Vitc
Nature's Most Important Dietary Supplement

Stephen R. Krauss, Ph.D.

Copyright ®2017
Oxigenesis, Inc.
Second Edition: First Printing 2017

ISBN: 978-1-5323-3029-2   Library of Congress

All rights reserved.
No part of this book may be reproduced in any form, except for the inclusion of brief quotations in a review or article, without the expressed written permission from the author.

Illustrations and cover artwork by Richard Shakelford.

Published by:
Oxigenesis, Inc. Paso Robles, CA 93446
805.549.0275 / fax 805.239.9790
e-mail: VitaminO@oxigenesis.com
website: http://www.oxigenesis.com

Printed in the U.S.A.

Author's Note:

The data and references provided and quoted in this book are based on research, experiments and information believed to be accurately and reliably reported for the applications described. However, no warranty is made, neither expressed nor implied, regarding the accuracy of the obtained results from the use of such data. The author will assume no responsibility for the results nor the performance of products and applications over which the author has no control.

The author has made every effort to keep the information as generic as possible by eliminating all references to trade-named products and has replaced all such names with the phrase "stabilized oxygen".

A glossary of many of the key concepts, terms and more technical words used in this book are found in Appendix One.

In Appendix Four you will find consumer and professional testimonials and comments about oxygen-based therapies and how they benefit the human body.

Acknowledgments:

This book is dedicated to my wife, Sherrie Lynn, for her continued faith, patience and counsel. Without her encouragement, I never would have devoted the time and energy into this project as well as investing my talents in the field of oxygen supplementation.

I would also like to thank Calvin Smith for sharing his wisdom and the numerous hours of stories that formed the real historical background for my search to find the truth about oxygen supplements. As a scientist, and a pioneer in this field, he was and will remain an inspiration to me.

Lastly, I would humbly like to thank the countless numbers of individuals who have allowed me into their personal lives during the last 40 years. They have willingly and honestly shared their health challenges and described how they benefitted from oxygen-based therapies. They remain the true pioneers in this field for they are the ones who have suffered greatly, never faltering in their hope to find relief from their infirmities.

Table of Contents

Foreword:	7
Introduction	11
Disclaimer	16
Chapter 1: An Introduction to Oxygen as a Nutritional Dietary Supplement	17
Chapter 2: The Blood Stream: The River of Life	27
Chapter 3: How Oxygen Kills Pathogens?	39
Chapter 4.: How Do Cells Create Their Energy	49
Chapter 5: When the Immune System Breaks Down	59
Chapter 6: Free Radicals: Enemies or Allies	65
Chapter 7: Oxygen & Muscle Basics	83
Chapter 8: Our Diet and Oxygen	101
Chapter 9: The Skin: Oxygen for the Body's Largest Organ	107
Chapter 10: Drugs, Disease & the Immune System	113
Chapter 11: Oxygen and the Brain	129
Chapter 12: Alternative Oxygen Therapies	137
Chapter 13: Hydrogen Peroxide Oxygen Therapy	149
Chapter 14: Ozone Therapies	157
Chapter 15: Hyperbaric Oxygen Therapies	161
Chapter 16: Oxygenated Bottled Water	167
Chapter 17: Stabilized Oxygen: Introducing Vitamin O	177
Chapter 18: Measuring the Energy Potential in Bottled Water	201
A Final Word from the Author	211
Appendix One: Oxygen and Nutritional Glossary	219
Appendix Two: For Further Study	253
Appendix Three: Dr. Otto Warburg, Ph.D. "On the Origin of Cancer Cells"	257
Appendix Four: Uses for Stabilized Oxygen	275
Appendix Five: Ozone: 150 years of Use	313

Foreward

Oxygen is the essential element for life on planet Earth. With the exception of a few small microbial organisms, all life requires this basic molecule to survive and proliferate. All plants and animals, both on land and in the oceans, utilize oxygen in order to convert fuel into energy. Without oxygen, which forms 21% of our planet's atmosphere, life as we know it would simply cease to exist.

From a human perspective, oxygen is the most important element which we take into our bodies. Aerobic metabolism, which uses oxygen to convert either carbohydrates or fats into energy, is the metabolic system keeping us alive. In the presence of oxygen, a single molecule of glucose can be fully metabolized to provide 32 molecules of energy in the form of ATP. The only by-products in this process are carbon dioxide and water; both of which can be easily removed from the body through expiration.

In the absence of oxygen, that same molecule of glucose only provides 2 molecules of energy. This form of metabolism produces lactic acid as a by-product which is one of the primary markers of peripheral fatigue. But more importantly, it is not economical enough to keep us alive for any length of time.

Clearly, therefore, oxygen is of huge importance for our health and wellbeing. In fact, one of the most accurate ways to predict how long a person will live, is to measure their body's ability to consume oxygen. Maximal oxygen consumption (VO_2max), calculated during an exercise test, is one of the strongest predictors of all-cause-mortality. A recent study by Ladenvall et al. (2016) reported that having a low VO_2max was strongly associated with an increased risk of death, even when other traditional risk factors such as smoking, high blood pressure and cholesterol were discounted. Furthermore, in a systematic review of obesity research, it was observed that aerobic fitness is a far stronger predictor of death than how overweight a person is (Barry et al., 2014). An obese individual has the same risk of death as a normal weight individual, as long as their maximal oxygen consumptions are matched. Perhaps, in our societal era of "body consciousness", we should care less about how we look in the mirror and more about how efficiently our bodies can consume oxygen.

In terms of human performance, the role which oxygen plays is equally as critical. Nowhere is this seen more clearly than when our bodies are starved of oxygen. Under normal conditions, oxygen passes efficiently from our lungs into our bloodstream. The hemoglobin in our blood has such a high affinity for oxygen that even during maximal intensity exercise, the blood leaving our lungs is almost completely saturated with oxygen. However, this affinity changes when we move to higher altitudes.

Once we reach a height in excess of 1,500 meters (5,000 feet), the air becomes too thin and oxygen can no longer bind effectively to hemoglobin. The higher we climb, fewer molecules of oxygen enter our bodies. Work becomes difficult, our breathing becomes labored, and we feel light-headed, often nauseous. These are the telltale signs of altitude sickness brought about by a lack of oxygen.

For the brave few climbers who dare to venture above the 8,000 meter barrier, known as the "death zone", the only way to survive for any length of time is to breathe supplemental oxygen. This approach has been shown to increase arterial oxygen saturation (Bannister & Cunningham, 1954), lower sub-maximal heart rate and blood lactate values (Asmussen & Nielsen, 1950), and increased maximal oxygen consumption or VO_2max.

In contrast to impaired human performance and increased fatigue in the absence of oxygen, there is a growing body of evidence supporting the enhancement of human performance by making oxygen more abundant using oxygen supplementation. Breathing air, with a higher than normal (21%) concentration of oxygen, has been shown to improve exercise tolerance (Oussaidene et al., 2013), sprint and endurance performance (Sperlich et al., 2011), and enhance recovery (Sperlich, Zinner, Hauser, Holmberg, & Wegrzyk, 2016). Therefore, by increasing the amount of oxygen circulating in our bodies, we improve our ability to perform.

The aim of this short foreword is to highlight how crucial oxygen is for both human performance and general wellbeing. It should also serve as a reminder of how important this molecule is to mankind, not to mention the multitude of other creatures that we share the planet with. We should be grateful to the forests and plains of the Earth for supplying this precious gift to us through the power of photosynthesis. Our very survival as a species depends on fully recognizing the importance of this gift and not squandering it through pollution and deforestation.

As you read this book, and learn more about the importance of oxygen for health and wellbeing, it is my hope that you will gain a greater appreciation of the Earth providing oxygen as gift to us, free of charge.

Neil Fleming, PhD.

References:
1. Asmussen, E., & Nielsen, M. (1950). The effect of autotransfusion of 'work blood' on the pulmonary ventilation. Acta Physiol Scand, 20, 79-87.
2. Bannister, R., & Cunningham, D. (1954). The effects of respiration and performance during exercise of adding oxygen to inspired air. . J Physiol, 125(118-137).
3. Barry, V. W., Baruth, M., Beets, M. W., Durstine, J. L., Liu, J., & Blair, S. N. (2014). Fitness vs. fatness on all-cause mortality: a meta-analysis. Prog Cardiovasc Dis, 56(4), 382-390. doi: 10.1016/j.pcad.2013.09.002

4. Ladenvall, P., Persson, C. U., Mandalenakis, Z., Wilhelmsen, L., Grimby, G., Svardsudd, K., & Hansson, P. O. (2016). Low aerobic capacity in middle-aged men associated with increased mortality rates during 45 years of follow-up. Eur J Prev Cardiol, 23(14), 1557-1564. doi: 10.1177/2047487316655466

5. Oussaidene, K., Prieur, F., Bougault, V., Borel, B., Matran, R., & Mucci, P. (2013). Cerebral oxygenation during hyperoxia-induced increase in exercise tolerance for untrained men. Eur J Appl Physiol, 113(8), 2047-2056. doi: 10.1007/s00421-013-2637-4

6. Sperlich, B., Zinner, C., Hauser, A., Holmberg, H. C., & Wegrzyk, J. (2016). The Impact of Hyperoxia on Human Performance and Recovery. Sports Med. doi: 10.1007/s40279-016-0590-1

7. Sperlich, B., Zinner, C., Krueger, M., Wegrzyk, J., Mester, J., & Holmberg, H. C. (2011). Ergogenic effect of hyperoxic recovery in elite swimmers performing high-intensity intervals. Scand J Med Sci Sports, 21(6), e421-429. doi: 10.1111/j.1600-0838.2011.01349.x

.

Neil Fleming holds a Ph.D. in Exercise Physiology and is currently a Postdoctoral Researcher at Trinity College, Dublin, Ireland. His expertise is in the TCD Human Performance Laboratory where his work focuses on the neuromuscular effects of exoskeletal walking and transcutaneous spinal stimulation in SCI (Spinal Chord Injury) patients. He teaches post-graduate studies in Exercise Physiology and Exercise Medicine. He was previously an Assistant Professor of Exercise Science at Indiana State University where he taught Exercise Science in Neuromuscular Physiology, Clinical Exercise Physiology and Coaching Science. Dr. Fleming has also conducted research in the role oxygen plays in human performance.

Introduction

> "Borel[1] makes the amusing supposition of a million monkeys allowed to play upon the keys of a million typewriters. What is the chance that this wanton activity should reproduce exactly all of the volumes which are contained in the library of the British Museum? It certainly is not a large chance, but it may be roughly calculated, and proves in fact to be considerably larger than the chance that a mixture of oxygen and nitrogen will separate into the two pure constituents. After we have learned to estimate such minute chances, and after we have overcome our fear of numbers which are very much larger or very much smaller than those ordinarily employed, we might proceed to calculate the chance of still more extraordinary occurrences, and even have the boldness to regard the living cell as a result of random arrangement and rearrangement of its atoms. However, we cannot but feel that this would be carrying extrapolation too far. This feeling is due not merely to a recognition of the enormous complexity of living tissue but to the conviction that the whole trend of life, the whole process of building up more and more diverse and complex structures, which we call evolution, is the very opposite of that which we might expect from the laws of chance."[2]
>
> Gilbert Newton Lewis[3]

Almost thirty years ago, I received a small sample bottle containing a solution that the inventor claimed would bring tremendous healing benefits to the body. I was told that the liquid contained a high concentration of "stabilized oxygen" which would not only destroy infectious microbes

---

[1] Félix Édouard Justin Émile Borel was a French mathematician and politician. As a mathematician, he was known for his founding work in the areas of measure theory and probability.

[2] The Anatomy of Science (1926), 158-9.

[3] Gilbert Newton Lewis (1875-1946) was an American physical chemist whose concept of electron pairs led to modern theories of chemical bonding. His concept of acids and bases was another fundamental contribution.

but would improve metabolism. I was both interested and a bit skeptical. I wanted to learn more.

Certainly oxygen is the key factor in sustaining life. But ingesting oxygen, and somehow having that same oxygen get into the blood stream, was another story altogether. Having spent as many years as I had in marketing and sales, one thing I knew was that product claims had to be substantiated by credible sources.

Getting my hands on detailed scientific information that described the "stabilizing" processes, analysis of chemical contents and studies demonstrating the efficacy of this and other oxygen-rich supplements, was nearly impossible. And so began my quest for the truth about stabilized oxygen which ultimately led me to conducting general research about oxygen and its function and importance to all living organisms.

Oxygen was independently discovered by the Swedish pharmacist Karl Scheele in 1772 and the English amateur chemist Joseph Priestly in 1775. Priestly called oxygen "dephlogisticated air" and after isolating it and breathing it he felt that it was "peculiarly beneficial." 236 years ago he wrote:

"Who can tell, but that, in time, this pure air may become a fashionable article in luxury. Hitherto, only two mice and myself have had the privilege of breathing it."[4]

From Priestly to today, thousands of articles have been written in publications, including medical journals, throughout the world describing oxygen's importance in maintaining and sustaining life. And yet, no other element has been

---

[4] Priestley, Joseph, LL.D. F.R.S. Experiments and Observations on Different Kinds of Air and Other Branches of Natural Philosophy Connected with the Subject (in three volumes). Printed by Thomas Pearson and Sold by J. Johnson, st. Paul's Church-Yard, London. MDCCXC.

surrounded with as much controversy. Life cannot exist without it and, because of its capacity to oxidize (or share electrons with virtually every other element that exists), oxygen does have a "darker side".

This book is not intended to be a science book, medical journal or compendium on oxygen and its medicinal use since oxygen was discovered back in 1772. It started out as a file of articles, studies and testimonials for my own personal use. But because the information was so diverse and, as I soon discovered, the facts surrounding oxygen therapies so misunderstood and misquoted, I soon discovered a growing need to put these materials in a book that was hopefully easy to read and understand.

The more I have learned about oxygen, its beneficial healing properties, its ability to cleanse, disinfect and improve health, the more I am convinced that it is not here on the earth by pure chance. There is a divinely inspired interaction between oxygen-producing plant life and oxygen-consuming higher life forms. A reduction in oxygen levels on our planet of even a few percentage points can adversely affect this delicate balance which maintains life or causes it to die out.

Only mankind, of all the thousands of species that exist, has the ability to drastically alter this balance. Certainly history has already shown that, because of our global irresponsibility, ignorance and complacency, we have already damaged the quality of the oxygen supply on this planet that we have been entrusted to protect.

Since the 1960s, the vision of our national spirit has been to "look to the stars". Space, and all the technology that embraces the realization of that dream, focuses on "outer space" or as the famous series Star Trek intoned: "the last frontier".

But the true mysteries of science, and the real "last" frontier for exploration, is "inner space" -- the human body, for it is the most complicated and miraculously designed biochemical marvel in all the visible universe, a universe that contains more than 100 billion galaxies, each with over 300 billion stars.

The human body has more than 37 trillion (not billion!) cells all originating from a single cell. This is the equivalent of the number of stars in 37,000 galaxies! And every single day more than 50 billion of our cells die and must be replaced.

We have more than 20 trillion red blood cells coursing through our bodies and more than 100 million are created in our bone marrow every single minute that we are alive. These red blood cells flow through an intricate labyrinth of blood vessels, capillaries and veins that is more than 100,000 miles long, (almost half the distance to the moon and more than four times around the circumference of the earth,) and our blood circulates this distance once every three minutes.

Inside every one of our cells is a human computer chip that stores everything about us in a twisted double helix of DNA that contains 440 million nucleotides, each containing about 30 atoms. This strand is only 6 microns across in size. (You need a high powered microscope just to see it.) Yet when stretched out, the DNA strand measures 2 meters (almost 6 feet) in length. In fact, if you were to stretch out all the DNA strands in every cell in our body, they would extend to twice the diameter of our solar system -- almost 15 billion miles long!)

To create every chemical bond, every new cell, every thought pattern or memory, requires a constant supply of the most important element on our planet: oxygen. You can go without food for 40 days, water for about seven days, but only a minute or two without life-giving oxygen.

Our communal desire to explore the fantastic mysteries of the human body and unravel the complexities of how this human-machine works and can be healed is worth our investments of time, energy and our resources.

Our mutual responsibility is greater than many imagine if we are to leave a legacy of clean air with healthy oxygen levels to our children and their children.

Stephen R. Krauss, Ph.D.
Paso Robles, California

Disclaimer

This book is based on a compilation and a summary of research that was conducted over a forty year period on a variety of stabilized oxygen supplements by professionals in numerous disciplines. This research was supplemented by dozens of studies conducted by independent testing laboratories, colleges and universities throughout the world.

The following information has been obtained by, or was provided to, the author both in written as well as verbal formats by individuals, testing facilities and consumers concerning their independent observations as to the benefits of stabilized oxygen products.

This information is not intended to recommend oxygen supplements as drugs, as a diagnosis for specific illnesses or conditions, nor as products to eliminate diseases or other medical conditions or complications. Rather, it is intended to provide an historical background on the combined data currently available on stabilized oxygen supplements.

The author makes no medical claims as to the benefits of stabilized oxygen to improve the medical condition of individuals. The author recommends that individuals always discuss their medical interests, diagnostic, or physiological concerns with a qualified physician or practitioner prior to purchasing and taking any oxygen-based supplement.

Please note that most stabilized oxygen supplements are normally sold as vitamin (dietary) supplements in the United States under the F.D.A.'s Dietary and Supplement Health Education Act (D.S.H.E.A.) and are not sold as prescription pharmaceuticals nor as over-the-counter drugs.

Chapter One:
An Introduction to Oxygen As a Nutritional Dietary Supplement

Oxidation is the source of life. Its lack causes impaired health or disease; its cessation, death.
Dr. Eugene Blass, Ph.D.[5]
Oxygen Therapy: Its Foundation, Aim and Result

For almost 250 years, researchers and health practitioners have observed that patients using oxygen-based therapies, (including stabilized oxygen supplements,) have experienced improved health and well-being.

The first recorded application of using oxygen in treating a patient occurred in 1783. This therapy was administered by the French physician Caillens.[6] Since that time, oxygen, as a therapeutic treatment, has been well researched and its benefits documented by thousands of experts in various medical and scientific disciplines.

Perhaps the most detailed chronological and annotated overview on "supplemental oxygen" therapies was compiled by Dr. Lawrence Martin, M.D., Chief, Division of Pulmonary and Critical Care Medicine at Mt. Sinai Medical Center in Cleveland, Ohio U.S.A. In his published article

---

[5] Dr. F. M. Eugene Blass, Ph.D., is also considered one of the fathers of oxygen therapy. In 1929, while looking for a cure for cancer, he developed what many claim to be the first powdered form of stabilized oxygen. Dr. Blass believed that a patient's bowel must be cleansed and free of any old impacted fecal matter (hardened mucus toxins) that might impair health. He realized that cancer and other pathogens did not live well in an oxygenated environment. Dr. Blass called his formula Homozone and it incorporated oxygen atoms bound to magnesium atoms. The product was designed to promote intestinal cleansing by eliminating accumulated hardened mucus waste.

[6] Martin, Dr. Lawrence, M.D. "Oxygen Therapy: The First 150 Years". Abstract. Mt. Sinai Medical Center, Cleveland, Ohio. Internet File. February, 1997.

"Oxygen Therapy: The First 150 Years", Dr. Martin wrote in his introduction:

> Although oxygen's life-supporting role was understood early on, it took about 150 years for the gas to be used in a proper fashion for patients. For the first 150 years after discovery, therapeutic use of oxygen was sporadic, erratic, controversial. comical, beset by quackery, and only occasionally helpful. Not until the pioneering work of Haldane, Stadie, Barcroft and others, early in the 20th century, was oxygen therapy placed on a rational, scientific basis.[7]

How can the most abundant element on the earth provide such remarkable physiological benefits? To answer this question, we first have to understand just what oxygen is and how important oxygen is to a healthy body.

Simple Oxygen Chemistry

Oxygen is one of the five basic elements of all life: oxygen, hydrogen, carbon, nitrogen and sulphur. It is colorless, tasteless and odorless. None of these five basic elements, or any other element for that matter, is as abundant on our earth as oxygen. In addition, only oxygen is capable of combining with almost every other element and it is essential in combustion, not only in the form that we call "fire", but also in generating the energy in every cell in our body.

The earth's crust is estimated to be 49.2% oxygen by weight; oxygen constitutes almost 85% of sea water, 47% of dry soil, 42% of all vegetation, 46% of igneous rocks and over 65% of the human body.

The two men credited with the discovery of oxygen in 1773 are the Swedish pharmacist Karl Wilhelm Scheele and English chemist Joseph Priestly. But it wasn't until 1777 that

---

[7] Ibid.

the French chemist and scientist Antoine Laurent Lavoisier demonstrated that oxygen was a pure substance and was a component of air.

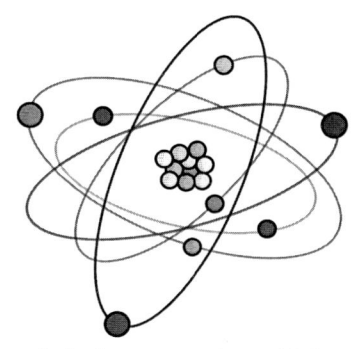

A single oxygen atom with its eight orbiting electrons.

The most common and stable form of oxygen is di-atomic oxygen, or "O_2". This is the primary molecular oxygen form used by all living creatures that is taken in during respiration. Other forms of oxygen, like singlet oxygen "O_1" and ozone "O_3", are more reactive and quickly combine with, or "oxidize", other atoms or molecules to form new compounds. It is oxygen's "reactive" nature that makes it so remarkable and beneficial.

Oxygen:
The Basis for All Life

No other element is as important as atomic oxygen (with its eight electrons per atom.) Oxygen is absolutely critical to the life processes of all living creatures. According to medical research, 90% of the aerobic metabolic energy we need in our bodies comes from aerobic metabolism linked to oxygen with only 10% of our energy coming from food.

Current scientific measurements of the air we breathe indicate that oxygen levels are about 20% by volume. The remainder of the gasses in our air is comprised of hydrogen, nitrogen, (the greatest component of air,) and other toxic and nontoxic gasses. Interestingly enough, some scientists believe that the levels of atmospheric oxygen were substantially higher when the earth was younger, as high as 50% according to some researchers. This theory has been debated for decades by the scientific community. Many of the experts content that:

> "Dinosaurs weren't done in by a giant asteroid, as one theory holds, but by a change in the atmosphere that meant there wasn't enough oxygen to support their inefficient respiratory systems..."[8]

Measurements of the oxygen levels in our air indicate that there has been a decline since the advent of the Industrial Revolution. Some medical professionals believe that the decline in atmospheric oxygen may be one of the causes of increased illness and the spread of many infectious diseases. (We will talk about oxygen's remarkable disinfecting power a bit later in the book.)

In the view of Hungarian Professor Dr. Ervin Laszlo, Ph.D., a drop in atmospheric oxygen has potentially serious physiological consequences.[9] Dr. Laszlo wrote:

---

[8] "Dinosaurs Weren't Done In By Asteroids", Associated Press Release, October 27, 1997.

[9] Dr. Laszlo, Founder and President of the Club of Budapest, is generally recognized as the founder of systems philosophy and general evolution theory. Formerly a Professor of Philosophy, Systems Science, and Futures Studies, Laszlo is the author or editor of 69 books translated into as many as 19 languages. He has also worked as Program Director for the United Nations Institute for Training and Research [UNITAR] and as President of the International Society for Systems Sciences. Currently, in addition to designing and overseeing the global projects of the Club of Budapest, he serves as Founder-Director of the General Evolution Research Group, Administrator of the Interdisciplinary University of Paris and other positions.

"Evidence from prehistoric times indicates that the oxygen content of pristine nature was above the 21% of total volume that it is today. It has decreased in recent times due mainly to the burning of coal in the middle of the last century. Currently the oxygen content of the Earth's atmosphere dips to 19% over impacted areas, and it is down to 12% to 17% over the major cities. At these levels it is difficult for people to get sufficient oxygen to maintain bodily health: it takes a proper intake of oxygen to keep body cells and organs, and the entire immune system, functioning at full efficiency. At the levels we have reached today cancers and other degenerative diseases are likely to develop. And at 6% to 7% life can no longer be sustained." [10]

Changes of the oxygen content in air that is breathed in, can cause the adverse physical reactions to the human body.

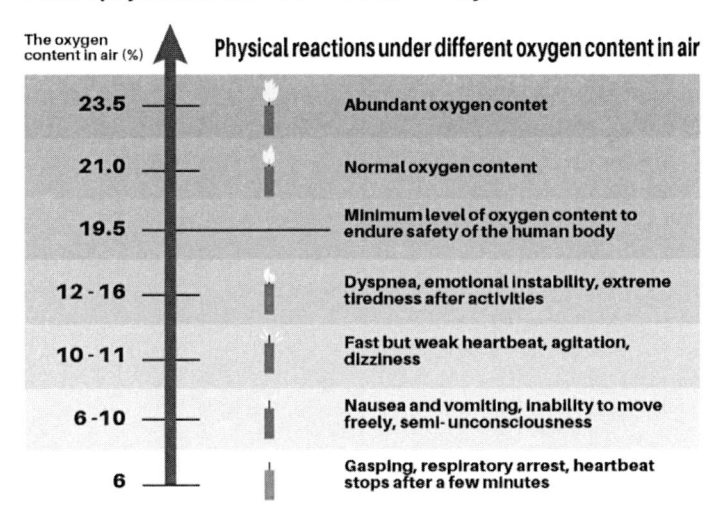

Physical reactions under different oxygen content in air

The oxygen content in air (%)	Physical reactions
23.5	Abundant oxygen contet
21.0	Normal oxygen content
19.5	Minimum level of oxygen content to endure safety of the human body
12 - 16	Dyspnea, emotional instability, extreme tiredness after activities
10 - 11	Fast but weak heartbeat, agitation, dizziness
6 - 10	Nausea and vomiting, inability to move freely, semi-unconsciousness
6	Gasping, respiratory arrest, heartbeat stops after a few minutes

---

[10] Thompson, Donald c., M.D. "Invisible Toxins Hurt the Immune System." Journal of Longevity Research, Vol3, No.5, 1997: 26-27.

Respiration

Oxygen is brought to the lungs by a process called "respiration" where oxygen (O_2) diffuses from the air into the blood stream through more than 140 square meters (about 460 square feet) of internal lung surface area. Each lung has over 300 million alveolar sacs which look like clusters or bunches of grapes. If these were flattened out and connected together they would make a surface area of about 260 square feet.

The average individual takes in approximately six liters (1.6 U.S. gallons) of air every minute, 757 liters (200 U.S. gallons) every hour. Under heavy exertion or stress, this rate will increase to as much as 15 liters (4 U.S. gallons) every minute. This oxygen from the lungs rapidly diffuses into the blood plasma as oxygen moves from the lungs' alveolar sacs and into the capillaries that surround these sacs. This is because the membranes of the alveoli are so thin that the oxygen molecules can pass right through them.

As these life-giving oxygen molecules diffuse into the blood stream, they bind to hemoglobin molecules in the iron-rich red blood cells. As the hemoglobin molecule accepts oxygen, it releases carbon dioxide which is released back out of the lungs as a waste gas. This exchange of gasses is what is called "respiration".

The hemoglobin molecules on each red blood cell become over 95% saturated with the available oxygen that dissolves into the blood stream. Once the oxygen attaches to these molecules, the oxygen is transported and then released to more than 100 trillion cells, 600 muscles, and 22 internal organs in our bodies. The oxygen, once in each cell, is consumed in a process that creates energy and heat. The more energy or warmth our body needs, the more oxygen that is consumed.

This process is called "oxidation" and carbohydrates (sugars), fats and proteins (substrates) are what are oxi-

Alveolar sacs in the lungs

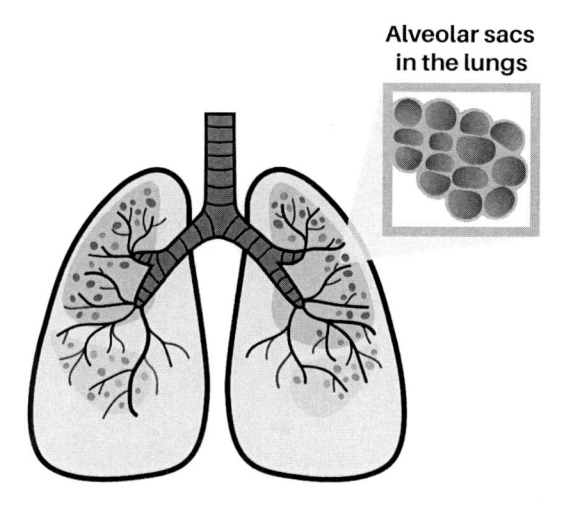

dized (or "burned") for the body's fuel. This process can only occur if a sufficient amount of oxygen is present.

For our cells to remain healthy and to continue to perform their functions of providing energy for the body, they must have an adequate and continuous supply of oxygen. It only makes sense that the lower the oxygen content of the body, the less the body is able to oxidize substrates for energy, reproduction and to detoxify itself.

Although oxygen is the substance that cells use in the greatest quantity, and on which all aerobic metabolism and cellular integrity depend, the tissues have no storage system for oxygen. They rely on a continuous supply of oxygen at a rate that precisely matches the body's changing metabolic requirements. If this oxygen supply fails, even for a few minutes, tissue hypoxaemia (oxygen tissue starvation) may develop resulting in anaerobic metabolism, (the production of lactic acid which causes pain,) cellular dysfunction and even cellular death.

Mineral deficiencies also contribute to oxygen depletion, especially a lack of iron, which is the only mineral whose sole function is to secure oxygen to each and every red blood cell. A lack of chromium affects blood sugar concentrations, and sugar (glucose) is essential in energy

Oxygenating the Red Blood Cell

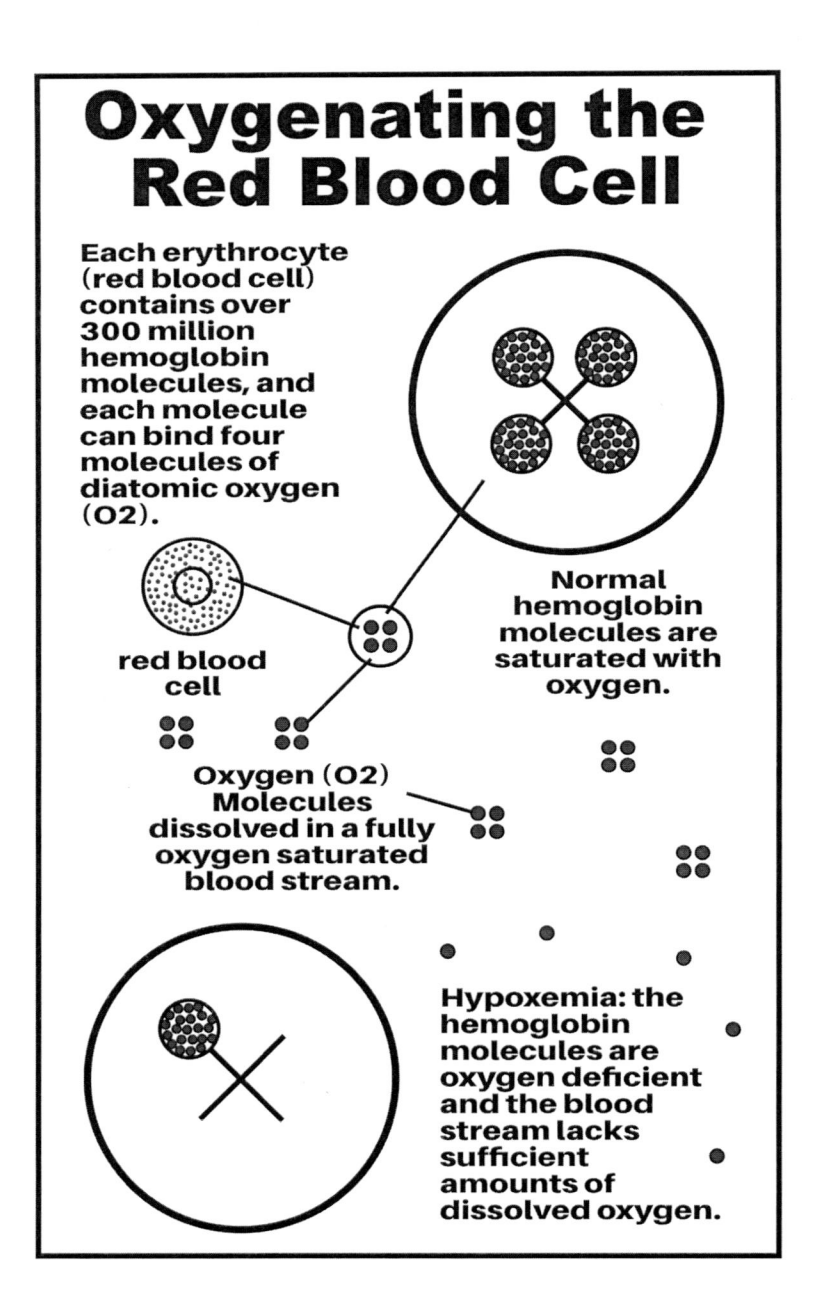

Each erythrocyte (red blood cell) contains over 300 million hemoglobin molecules, and each molecule can bind four molecules of diatomic oxygen (O_2).

red blood cell

Normal hemoglobin molecules are saturated with oxygen.

Oxygen (O_2) Molecules dissolved in a fully oxygen saturated blood stream.

Hypoxemia: the hemoglobin molecules are oxygen deficient and the blood stream lacks sufficient amounts of dissolved oxygen.

production. Cobalt is important to red blood cell reproduction. Copper is required as a catalyst to store and release iron. Magnesium and phosphorus are also involved in energy production. Manganese is a key component of every oxygen-handling enzyme.

Many foods form acids in the body and may temporarily reduce our oxygen and mineral reserves. These include flesh foods (primarily red meats), refined grains, soft drinks, carbonated drinks and alcoholic beverages.

Remember that the major function of the circulatory system is to transport oxygen from the lungs to the tissues at a rate that satisfies overall oxygen consumption by the cells and organs, including the brain which uses more than 25% of all the oxygen we breathe. A failure to supply sufficient oxygen to meet the metabolic requirements of the cells results in circulatory shock.

Under normal conditions, the total or "global" oxygen delivery (DO_2) is more than adequate to meet the total tissue oxygen requirements (VO_2) for aerobic metabolism. But, under prolonged stress and illness, this ratio is significantly lowered.

Do we get enough oxygen into our blood stream? And if we do not, what happens to our cells and vital organs when they are denied an adequate supply of oxygen? These are vital questions that scientists and researchers have debated for many years. At the heart of their search for answers is the intricate and important functioning of the blood stream, the "river of life", which is the transportation system for nutritional oxygen.

Chapter 2:
The Blood Stream: The River of Life

Oxygen is needed in the body. We can be without food and water for a lengthy time. We can be without oxygen only for a few seconds. It is the spark of life.
Dr. Charles H. Farr, M.D.,Ph.D.[11]
O2 Therapies

The average adult has about five liters (1.3 U.S. gallons) of blood inside of his or her body, coursing through the blood vessels, delivering essential elements, oxygen, and removing harmful wastes. Without blood, the human body would simply stop working.

Blood is the fluid of life, transporting oxygen from the lungs to the body tissue and transporting carbon dioxide as a waste product of metabolism from body tissues back to the lungs. Blood is the fluid of growth, delivering nourishment from digestion and hormones from the glands throughout the body. Blood is also the fluid of health, providing a highway for disease fighting substances and white blood cells to the tissues and removing wastes from the kidneys.

Because the blood stream contains living cells, our blood is "alive". Red blood cells and white blood cells are responsible for nourishing and cleansing the body and these blood cells have a life cycle, just as all living organisms do. Since the cells are alive, they too need nourishment. Oxygen, vitamins and minerals keep the blood healthy.

Human blood has three major components: the plasma, white blood cells and red blood cells. Blood will

---

[11] Charles H. Farr, MD, PhD (1927-1998) is often referred to as the "Father of Oxidative Medicine." He discovered "a positive metabolic effect to intravenous infusions of hydrogen peroxide," and authored a book on the subject.

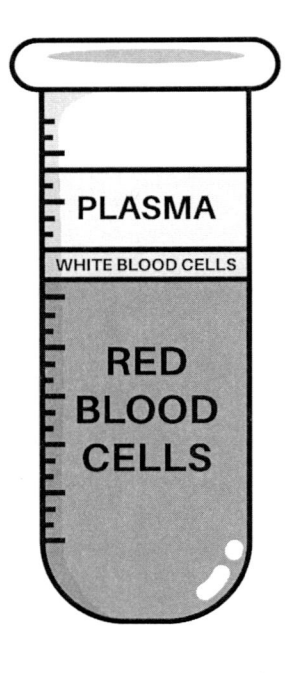

settle into these three distinct layers if left in a test tube. The red blood cells, the most numerous in the blood stream, will settle on the bottom. White blood cells, including lymphocytes, monocytes, eosinophils, basophils, neutrophils, and platelets, will form a thin white line in the middle. The deep-yellow and watery plasma will float to the top.

Of the three components, the plasma is the actual "river" in which all the working constituents of our blood are carried in our remarkable circulatory system. Among the many constituents in this river is dissolved oxygen, (up to 3% can be dissolved in this fluid,) minerals, vitamins, carbohydrates, amino acids and enzymes. Unlike fish that can exist only on the dissolved oxygen in their plasma stream, the human body requires more oxygen than the plasma can provide.

Red Blood Cells

Red blood cells perform the most important blood duty. A single drop of blood contains millions of red blood cells that are constantly traveling through the body delivering oxygen and removing wastes. If they failed to complete these tasks, the body would slowly die.

Red blood cells are red only because they contain a protein chemical called hemoglobin, which is bright red in color. Hemoglobin contains the element Iron, making it an excellent vehicle for transporting oxygen and carbon dioxide. As blood passes through the lungs, oxygen molecules attach to the hemoglobin. As the blood passes through the body's tissues, the hemoglobin releases the oxygen to the cells. The empty hemoglobin molecules then bond with

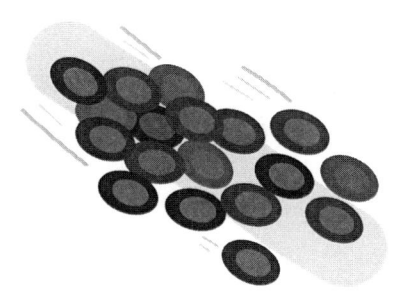

Red blood cells transport life-giving oxygen to trillions of cells every second we are alive.

carbon dioxide transporting this waste gas away from the cells and back to the lungs to be expelled.

Over time, the red blood cells get worn out and eventually die. In fact, the average life cycle of a red blood cell is 120 days. Fortunately, our bone marrow continually produces new blood cells, replenishing our supply.

The human heart beats about 100,000 times in a day. As mentioned previously, a normal human body has about 5 liters of total blood volume and a normal heart pumps blood at about 5 liters per minute. A red blood cell can leave the heart and travel down the leg and circle the toe and then return through the veins back to the heart in a round trip that will normally take no more than three minutes, depending on the health of the cardiovascular system. That is a total distance of about twelve feet traveled in three minutes, which is four feet per minute or more than 240 miles per hour. As one physician wrote:

> *"But there is truly a wide range of blood velocities throughout the body, even in a healthy person. Blood normally rushes through your brain and kid-*

neys at breakneck speed, but travels very slowly through your muscles when you are sedentary. (This is why you get up and stretch, so you can return all of that stagnant pooled blood to your heart and circulation.) The very fastest velocity that a given red cell experiences is when it is exiting the heart during a ventricular contraction. Whoosh...it leaves the heart at several feet per second, and the slowest velocity is nearly zero, when your stagnant blood is pooling in your extremities."[12]

Red Blood Types:

Everybody's blood is not the same. There are actually four different blood types. In addition, all blood has Rh factors that make it even more unique and distinct from someone else's blood. This is why blood received through a transfusion must match our own.

Yet, in some ways, every person's blood is the same. It is only when analyzed under a microscope that distinct differences are visible. In the early 20th century, an Austrian scientist named Karl Landsteiner was the first to classify blood according to those differences. He was awarded the Nobel Prize for his achievements. Landsteiner observed two distinct chemical molecules present on the surface of the red blood cells. He labeled one molecule "A" and the other molecule "B." If the red blood cell had only "A" molecules on it, that blood was called Type A. If the red blood cell had only "B" molecules on it, that blood was called Type B. If the red blood cell had a mixture of both molecules, that blood was called Type AB. If the red blood cell had neither molecule, that blood was called Type O.

If two different blood types are mixed together, the blood cells begin to clump together in the blood vessels, causing a potentially fatal situation. This is why it is impor-

---

[12] Starr, Sonya c., B.S., N.C. "Oxygen - 02: The Life Giving Element." The Nutrition & Dietary Consultant, August 1986.

tant that blood types be matched before blood transfusions take place. In an emergency, type O blood can be given because it is most likely to be accepted by all blood types.

A person with Type A blood can donate blood to a person with Type A or Type AB. A person with Type B blood can donate blood to a person with Type B or Type AB. A person with Type AB blood can donate blood to a person with Type AB only. A person with Type O blood can donate to anyone. A person with Type A blood can receive blood from a person with Type A or Type O. A person with Type B blood can receive blood from a person with Type B or Type O. A person with Type AB blood can receive blood from anyone. A person with Type O blood can receive blood only from a person with Type O. Because of these patterns, a person with Type O blood is said to be a universal donor. A person with Type AB blood is said to be a universal receiver.

Blood Donors

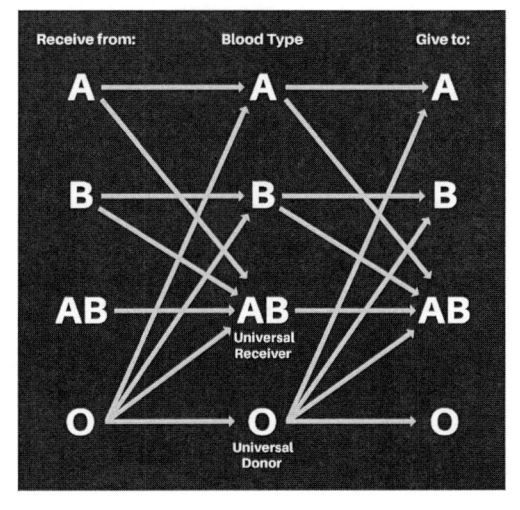

Receive from:	Blood Type	Give to:
A	A	A
B	B	B
AB	AB (Universal Receiver)	AB
O	O (Universal Donor)	O

The four main types of human blood and to whom each can contribute blood as well as from home blood can be accepted. Type AB is considered the Universal Receiver and Type O is the Universal Donor.

Red blood cells are important because their role is to carry tremendous amounts of oxygen to the tissues in our bodies. But these red blood cells also get some of their oxygen from the plasma. The body, in its own remarkable way, does not allow all of the red blood cells' oxygen to be consumed as it courses through our bodies. Under normal conditions, 70% to 75% of the oxygen that starts the journey in the red cells completes the return trip to the lungs. If, however, the body undergoes exertion, stress, illness or any other prolonged physical activity, this "reserve" can drop to 20% to 25%.

Dr. Arthur Guyton, M.D., author of the most widely accepted textbook on medical physiology, wrote:

> *"Normally, about 97% of the oxygen transported from the lungs to the tissues is carried in chemical combination with hemoglobin in the red blood cells, and the remaining three percent in the dissolved state in the water of the plasma and the cells...The fraction of the blood that gives up its oxygen as it passes through the tissue capillaries is called the utilization coefficient. Normally, this is approximately 0.25, or 25% of the blood...During strenuous exercise, as much as 75% to 85% of the blood can give up its oxygen...However, in local tissue areas where the blood flow is very slow or the metabolic rate very high, utilization coefficients approaching 100% have been recorded -- that is, essentially all the oxygen is removed."*[13]

It seems obvious that, if you can raise the amount of oxygen dissolved in the plasma, primarily at the lung alveolar interface, as well as at other sites, you will also increase the amount of oxygen that gets to the cells and that can become a part of the oxygen "reserve". (Keep this principle

---

[13] Guyton, Arthur C. The Textbook of Medical Physiology, (5th Edition) Pennsylvania:WB Saunders Co., 1976.

in mind as we discuss oxygen supplements later in the book.) The red blood cells, as carriers or the transportation system for oxygen, gather oxygen from the plasma and deliver this much needed oxygen to the capillaries where it is released again into the plasma for the cells to use to create the energy they need for healthy cellular metabolism.

White Blood Cells:

Whenever a germ or infection enters the body, the white blood cells snap to attention and race toward the "scene of the crime". The white blood cells are continually on the lookout for signs of disease. When a germ does appear, the white blood cells have a variety of ways by which they can attack. Some will produce protective antibodies that will overpower the germ. Others will surround and devour the invader.

White blood cells have a rather short life cycle, living from a few days to just a few weeks. A drop of blood can contain anywhere from 7,000 to 25,000 white blood cells at a time. If an invading infection fights back and persists, that number will significantly increase. A consistently high number of white blood cells is a symptom of Leukemia, a cancer of the blood. (A Leukemia patient may have as many as 50,000 white blood cells in a single drop of blood.)

White blood cells, also called "Leukocytes" are an important part of the body's immune system. They help prevent and fight infections. There are three main types of white blood cells: Monocytes, Granulocytes and Lymphocytes, each with an important role in fighting infections.

Monocytes are the largest of the white blood cells and make up from three to eight per cent of the total white blood cell volume. When monocytes leave the blood stream and enter our tissues or organs, they evolve into larger cells called macrophages that have an increased ability to destroy foreign organisms invading the body.

Granulocytes are any one of several types of white blood cells whose interior liquid contains granules that contain enzymes that are capable of killing microorganisms and breaking down the debris that is ingested by the cells. Granulocytes include the Neutrophil, the Eosinophil and Basophil cells.

The Neutrophil is the most abundant and important of these three immune cells making up 50% to 70% of the total white cell count. Neutrophils are phagocytic, which means they gobble up any foreign bacteria they come across.

A Lymphocyte is one of the nearly colorless cells of the blood and lymphatic system. It is produced in the bone marrow as well as in the lymph nodes and thymus gland. Lymphocytes have a nucleus and are chiefly responsible for maintaining our immunity to disease. These cells defend the body against infection by producing antibodies or toxic substances that destroy viruses and other foreign bodies. B cells and T cells are two types of Lymphocytes .

The T–cell is an abbreviation for T-Lymphocyte Cell. It is a white blood cell that makes its way through the body to the Thymus gland, which is located in the chest cavity. In the thymus these white cells mature into T-cells. From there, the T-cells circulate in the blood, spleen and particularly the lymph glands. T-cells provide protection against certain bacteria, viruses, and other disease-causing organisms that have already infected a cell and are growing inside the cells of the body. As these foreign bodies inside our cells multiply or cause damage, they are hidden from the antibodies made by the white B-cells. But the T-cells can recognize an infected cell and will attack it and destroy the hidden intruder.

T-cells work together with the B-cells and the Macrophages during an immune defense response. T-cells attract Macrophages to the intruder and stimulate the process called "phagocytosis". (Phagocytosis is a method T-cells use to surround and engulf diseased cells or invading pathogens, just as an amoeba would do.) In addition, B-cells produce more antibodies when T cells are present.

THE PROCESS OF PHAGOCYTOSIS

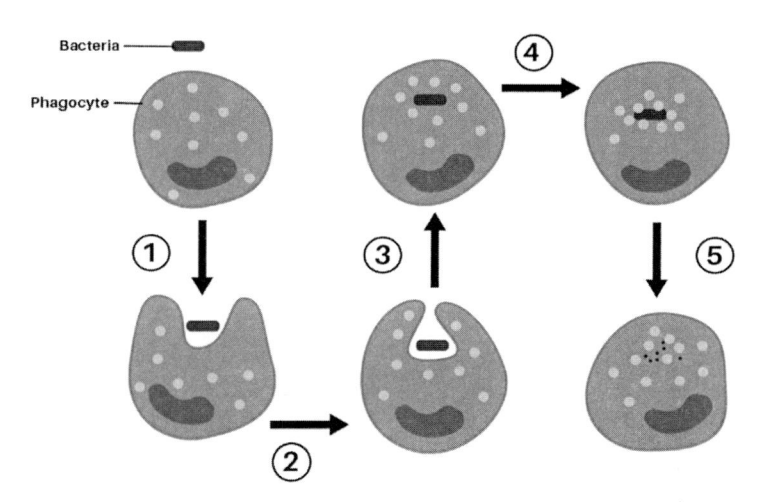

A white blood cell (T-cell) attacking an invading pathogen in the process called "phagocytosis". At the end of Stage 1, the white blood cell (phagocyte) extends to arms (pseudopodia) outward to surround the pathogen. At Stage 2 the pathogen is completely engulfed by the pseudopodia. In Stage 3, the pathogen is ingested. In Stage 4, the phagocyte releases lysosomal enzyme bursts containing high levels of oxygen in the form of hydrogen peroxide (H_2O_2). In Stage 4, the H_2O_2 breaks down into oxygen free radicals that attack and degrade the pathogen into small fragments.

T-cells are divided into four major groups

Not all T-cells are alike. T-cells, also called TH, T4 or CD4 cells, help other cells destroy infectious organisms. They are more like a "private investigator" because they do not attack invading microorganisms but rather decide whether an organism is a threat and whether the body should turn on its immune system. Helper T-cells can order B-cells into action. They point out foreign antigens to the B-cells which in turn manufacture a "Y" shaped protein called an "immunoglobulin" or "antibody". This antibody zeroes in on the antigen and attaches to the surface of the invading cell, killing it.

Suppressor T-cells, also called TS, T8 or CD8 cells, like Helper T-cells, do not attack invading microorganisms. Their job is to switch off both the B and T Lymphocytes attack when an infection has stopped and recovery is complete so that the aggressive T-cells don't destroy normal tissue.

Killer T-Cells, also called cytotoxic T Lymphocytes, or CTLs, recognize and destroy abnormal or infected cells in the body once Killer T-cells have received permission from the Helper T-cells. Most of the body's white cells will recognize other normal body cells and will leave them alone. But with the assistance of Helper T-cells, Killer T-cells seek out and destroy any of the body cells that have hidden microorganisms inside of them. Killer T-cells use a very strong enzyme, which contains oxygen as it's killing agent, against infected cells to destroy them. The action of Killer-T cells stimulates an increase in Macrophage activity which in turn cleans up the debris.

Natural Killer Cells (NK) cells are actually primitive T-cells that are free to attack indiscriminately without requiring permission from a Helper T-cell. This makes them the immune system's first line of defense. Since they lack receptors for identifying antigens, NK cells work best when their target has first been identified by macrophages and Helper T-cells.

Helper cells cells release the chemical messenger interferon which attracts and stimulates NK cells, causing them to grow larger and more aggressive. NK cells also zero in readily on targets that have already been coated with antibodies, such as tumor cells and body cells infected with a

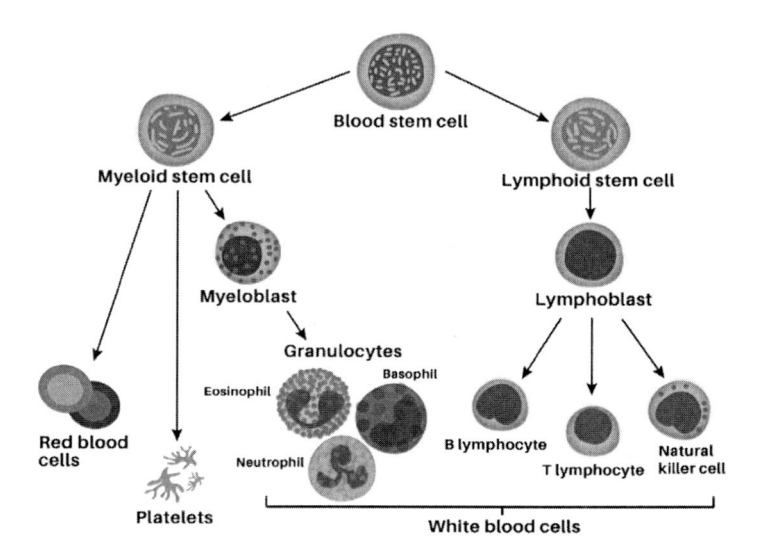

It is remarkable how many different cells evolve from a stem cell. What types of cells we need, at any given moment, are determined in a yet to be fully understood signaling system in the brain.

virus. NK cells swiftly migrate through the bloodstream and immediately kill with their oxygen-based toxic enzymes.

This may all seem very complex and overwhelming to understand. But the great news is that our bodies know exactly what type of white blood cells we need at any location and at any instant of time. Our white blood cells are on guard to protect us against invading organisms ever second of every minute we are alive. These are the tactical special forces of our standing army using oxygen as their most lethal weapon against an ever evolving invading force that has no other purpose than to overwhelm us with their numbers and take over our metabolic activity.

Chapter 3:
How oxygen kills pathogens

The fungus is knocking out species...It impedes the ability of the skin to absorb oxygen and just suffocates them. It's the equivalent of us ingesting a fungus that takes over our lungs.
Dr. Claude Gascon, Ph.D.[14]

    Higher life forms depend on oxygen to create energy for the cells. But there are unicellular microorganisms that fear oxygen because of its ability to also destroy life. This process is called "oxidation" and relies on oxygen's unique ability to attract (or "receive") electrons from other atoms and molecules.
    Surrounding the nucleus of atoms are electrons that spin in orbits. When an orbit lacks a set of "paired electrons", that orbit will make every effort to attach itself to another atom, or group of atoms, so that the orbiting electrons become more stable. These atoms may even "steal" electrons from other atoms or molecules. (Molecules are a group of two or more atoms jointed together).
    To help visualize the remarkable potential of electrons, imagine yourself spinning a golf ball around yourself and that this golf ball is connected to a spring. The golf ball represents an electron and the place where you are standing is where the atom's nucleus would be. If you spin the golf ball around you in a constant speed, the electron will be at the same distance from you, spinning at the same speed you are turning. If you start to spin harder, by putting more energy into your spin, the golf ball will move away from you and the spring will expand. Likewise, if you spin more slowly,

---

[14] Dr. Claude Gascon, Ph.D. is the Senior Vice President and Chief Science Officer at the National Fish and Wildlife Foundation. The National Fish and Wildlife Foundation (NFWF) protects and restores our nation's wildlife and habitats. Chartered by Congress in 1984, NFWF directs public conservation dollars to the most pressing environmental needs.

the golf ball will be closer to you and the spring will contract. In the same way, with changes in energy, an electron can occupy a different orbit around its nucleus.

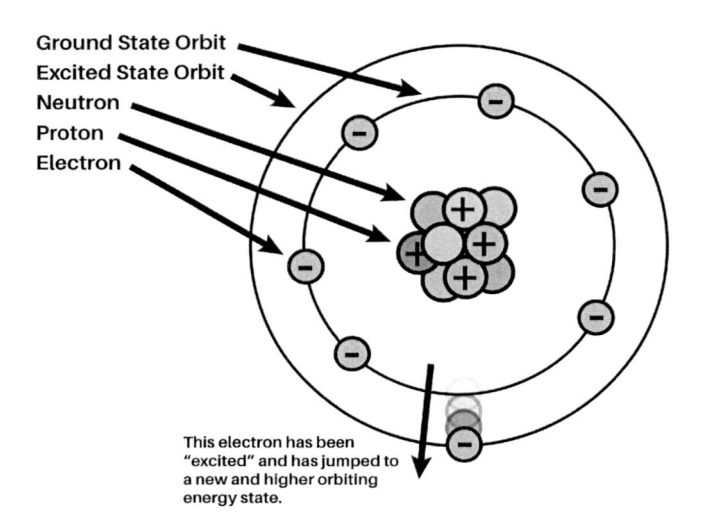

Ground State Orbit
Excited State Orbit
Neutron
Proton
Electron

This electron has been "excited" and has jumped to a new and higher orbiting energy state.

The smallest of these orbits represents the lowest energy that the electron can possess. This lowest energy state is known as the "ground state." If the electron absorbs energy of the right amount, (such as visible light, infrared heat, or ultraviolet light,) the electron can jump to a higher orbit or "energy level" in the atom. With the electron in a higher orbit, the atom is said to be in the "excited state." At this point, the electron can fall back to a lower energy orbit or even the ground state. As it falls one orbit at a time, it emits a certain amount of energy, which may also be in the form of light, heat, or so on.

It is the remarkable movement, and the exchange of electrons on an atomic and subatomic basis, that actually serves as a defense mechanism for our immune system. It is also a process to control the dangerous microorganisms that cause every known disease on the planet today.

How Unicellular Organisms React to the Presence of Oxygen:

Unicellular (single cell) microorganisms fall into four general categories that describe how these microbes react to the presence of oxygen: aerobes, aerotolerant anaerobes, strict anaerobes and facultative anaerobes.

AEROBES are microorganisms that require the presence of oxygen to live and reproduce themselves. Strict aerobes cannot survive in the absence of oxygen and produce energy only by oxidative phosphorylation[15].

AEROTOLERANT ANAEROBES are microorganisms that do not require the presence or oxygen to live and reproduce, and are not destroyed if oxygen is present. They generate energy only by fermentation and have mechanisms to protect themselves from oxygen.

STRICT ANAEROBES, in most cases, generate their energy by fermentation or by anaerobic respiration and are always killed in the presence of oxygen. These organisms are also called "obligate anaerobes". Obligate anaerobes vary greatly in their sensitivity to oxygen. Extremely oxygen-sensitive anaerobes, such as spirochetes[16] and some Clostridium species, cannot tolerate even 0.5% oxygen. Thus, oxygen is always toxic for them.

---

[15] Oxidative phosphorylation is a biochemical process in cells. It is the final metabolic pathway of cellular respiration in which energy, as ATP, is created in the cell's mitochondria.

[16] Spirochetes are long and slender bacteria, usually only a fraction of a micron in diameter, between 5 to 250 microns in size. They are tightly coiled and look like miniature springs. Members of this group are also unusual among bacteria because of the arrangement of axial filaments, which are otherwise similar to bacterial flagella, that enable the bacterium to move by rotating in place. Spirochetes include both syphilis and Lyme disease.

FACULTATIVE ANAEROBES prefer to grow in the presence of oxygen, using oxidative phosphorylation, but can also grow in an anaerobic environment using fermentation. The most virulent and destructive pathogens that affect mankind generally fall into the "strict anaerobe" category. They include bacteria like Staphylococcus aureus, Streptococcus pneumoniae, Clostridium botulinum and Escherichia coli. Viruses include Mycobacterium bovis, Herpesviridae and Influenza A virus/Orthomyxoviridae.

Oxygen has a tendency to form very reactive by-products, including hydrogen peroxide (H_2O_2) and O_2-superoxide, inside a cell. These by-products create havoc by reacting with proteins and cellular DNA, changing and/or destroying them.

Cells that are able to live in the presence of oxygen have enzymes, (like Superoxide Dismutase, Catalase and Peroxidase,) that help them cope with H_2O_2 and O_2^- and so are not destroyed by the presence of oxygen.

Unfortunately, oxygen's antimicrobial mechanisms are not completely understood. It is known that the cellular envelopes surrounding many anaerobic pathogens, like bacteria, are made up of polysaccharides, enzymes and proteins. In gram-negative[17] pathogenic organisms, fatty acid alkyl chains and helical lipoproteins are present. In acid-

---

[17] The phrase "gram negative" or "gram-positive" is a term used by microbiologists to classify bacteria into two groups. This positive/negative reference is based on the bacterium's chemical and physical cell wall properties. Gram-positive bacteria have a very thick cell wall made of a protein called peptidoglycan. These bacteria retain a crystal violet dye (stain). Gram-negative bacteria have a very thin peptidoglycan layer that is sandwiched between an inner cell membrane and a bacterial outer membrane and retain the pink dye. Usually, gram-positive bacteria are the helpful probiotic bacteria found in our digestive tract. Gram-negative bacteria are usually the ones that are harmful and include several species of Escherichia coli (E. coli), the common cause of food-borne disease and Vibrio cholera, the waterborne pathogen bacteria responsible for cholera.

fast[18] bacteria, such as Mycobacterium tuberculosis, one third to one half of the capsule is composed of complex lipids, (which are esterified mycolic acid, in addition to normal fatty acids), and glycolipids (sulfolipids, lipopolysaccharides, mycosides, trehalose mycolates).

It is the high lipid content of the cellular wall structure of these pathogenic organisms that may explain their sensitivity, and eventual destruction, when exposed to oxygen molecules. Oxygen breaks the chemical bonds in the molecules that make up the cell walls. It is like punching a hole in a dam. The pressure from the inside against the walls is great enough to cause what is inside to be forced outside. Oxygen disorganizes cellular membrane permeability so that the organism's nucleic acids and other components leak out and so the cell dies.

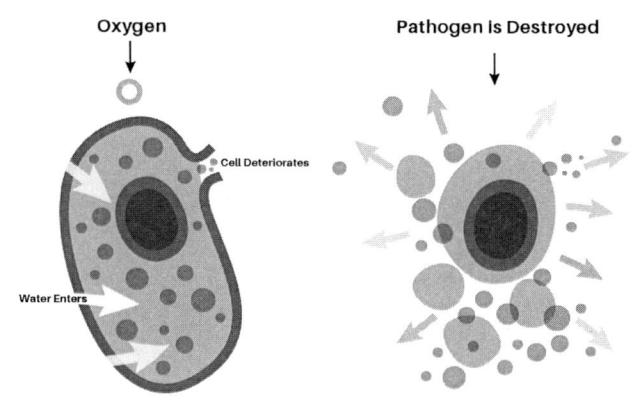

Oxygen molecules attack and destroy the cellular membranes of pathogenic microorganisms causing them to disintegrate.

---

[18] The acid-fast stain is a differential stain used to identify acid-fast organisms such as members of the genus Mycobacterium. Acid-fast organisms are characterized by wax-like, nearly impermeable cell walls. They contain mycolic acid and large amounts of fatty acids, waxes, and complex lipids. Acid-fast organisms are highly resistant to disinfectants and dry conditions. Because the cell wall is so resistant to most compounds, acid-fast organisms require a special staining technique. The primary stain used in acid-fast staining, carbolfuchsin, is lipid-soluble and contains phenol, which helps the stain penetrate the cell wall.

Oxygen molecules easily penetrate these cellular envelopes and affect the cytoplasmic integrity of pathogenic organisms. In addition, oxygen disrupts the metabolic activity of these disease-causing cells.

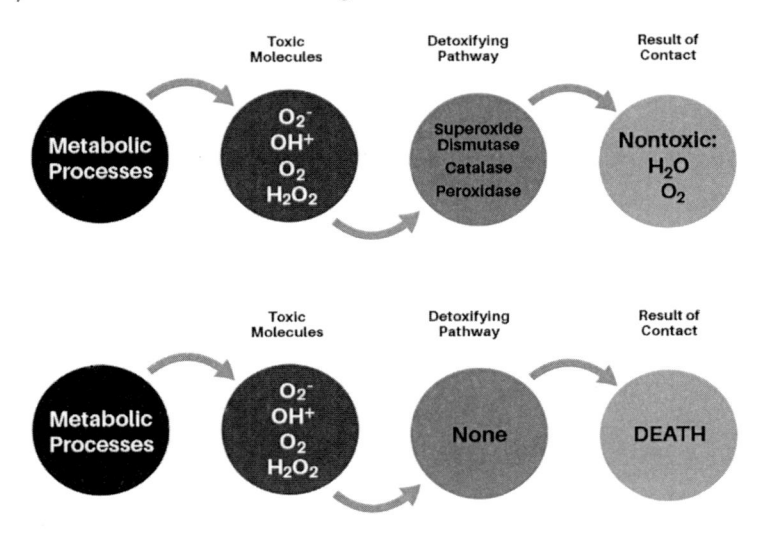

	Toxic Molecules	Detoxifying Pathway	Result of Contact
Metabolic Processes	O_2^-, OH^+, O_2, H_2O_2	Superoxide Dismutase, Catalase, Peroxidase	Nontoxic: H_2O, O_2
Metabolic Processes	O_2^-, OH^+, O_2, H_2O_2	None	DEATH

Oxygen destroys pathogens in a number of different ways: oxygen short-circuits the processes by which pathogens create energy; oxygen disturbs the structure of the bacterial cell wall; oxygen also interferes with the production of essential proteins.

TOP (above): Aerobic organisms possess enzymes that deactivate oxygen so that reactive toxic molecules containing oxygen do not damage the cells.

BOTTOM (above): Unlike aerobic organisms, anaerobic organisms do not possess enzymes that are able to deactivate oxygen. Thus, reactive toxic molecules containing oxygen, damage the cells' structural integrity, stop the metabolic processes, and bring about cellular destruction and death.

Oxygen also exchanges atoms and electrons with other compounds, such as the enzymes, lipids, etc. in these organisms. When enzymes come in contact with oxygen, one or more of the hydrogen atoms in the molecules are replaced by oxygen. This causes the entire molecule to change shape or fall apart. When enzymes do not function properly, a microorganism will die.

So, oxygen disrupts the integrity of the bacterial cell envelope through oxidation of the phospholipids and lipoproteins. In fungi, oxygen inhibits cell growth at a number of stages. With viruses, oxygen damages the viral capsid and disrupts the reproductive cycle. The weak enzyme coatings on cells that make them vulnerable to invasion by viruses also make them susceptible to oxidation and elimination from the body, which then replaces them with healthy cells.

The Body's Immune System Defends Itself with Oxygen:

The body's immune system utilizes oxygen's powerful oxidizing potential on pathogens in another remarkable way. When a pathogen infects the body, the body recognizes this invasion and, as was previously explained, sends a host of warrior Phagocyte cells to attack and destroy this unwanted guest.

When a pathogen is in close proximity to a Phagocyte, some sort of signal, (the nature of which is still not clearly understood,) triggers the phagocyte digestion (ingestion) process. Ingestion involves the encircling of the target pathogen with the phagocytic membrane so that the pathogen is actually taken inside the cytoplasm of the phagocyte. It is engulfed in a membrane vesicle called a phagosome.

This process requires ATP (adenosine triphosphate), energy created by "oxygen". Contact between a pathogen and a Phagocyte also changes the phagocyte's metabolism from an aerobic respiratory process to anaerobic fermentative process, with lactic acid being the final end product. This increase in lactic acid in the Phagocyte lowers the pH of the cytoplasm, including the phagolysosome, and this enhances the activity of many of the enzymes present.

The phagosome, containing the microorganism, migrates into the cytoplasm and soon collides with a series of lysosomes and forms a phagolysosome. When the membranes of the phagosome and lysosome meet, the contents of the lysosome explosively discharge, releasing a large number of toxic reactive oxygen macromolecules (free radicals), as well as other compounds, into the phagosome. The killing processes inside the phagolysosome are confined to the organelle of the phagolysosome, and this protects the cytoplasm of the phagocyte from these toxic activities.

Several minutes after phagolysosome formation, the first detectable effect on the microorganism is that it loses its ability to reproduce. Inhibiting macromolecular synthesis occurs sometime later and most pathogenic organisms are dead 10 to 30 minutes after ingestion.

All anaerobic pathogens are rendered harmless in the presence of oxygen. The following is a description of some of the most common, and some of the most dangerous, organisms that attack and destroy the human body and which, by the way, oxygen instantly kills.

Numerous families of viruses, including Poliovirus 1 and 2, Human Rotaviruses, Norwalk virus, Parvoviruses, and Hepatitis A, B, and non-A non-B (C), among many others, are adversely affected by the presence of oxygen molecules. Most research on oxygen's virucidal effects appear to indicate that oxygen breaks apart the lipid molecules at the sites of multiple bond configurations. Once the virus' lipid envelop is fragmented, the cell's DNA or RNA is then quickly destroyed.

Non-enveloped viruses, including Adenoviridae, Picornaviridae, Coxsachie, Echovirus, Rhinovirus, Hepatitis A and E, and Reoviridae (Rotavirus), are viruses that do not have traditional cell envelopes and so are called "naked viruses." They have a nucleic acid core, made of DNA or RNA, and a nucleic acid coat, or "capsid", which is made of protein. Oxygen not only reacts with unsaturated lipids, it can also interact with proteins and protein constituents, especially amino acids. When oxygen contacts capsid proteins, protein hydroxides and protein hydroperoxides are formed.

Normal mammalian[19] cells possess a complex system of enzymes (including superoxide dismutase, catalase, peroxidase) which tend to ward off the effects of free radical oxygen species. Virus pathogens have no such protection against oxidative stress and are devoid of similar defensive mechanisms. Oxygen's effect upon cellular unsaturated lipids is only one of its documented biochemical actions. Oxygen is known to interact with the proteins, carbohydrates, and nucleic acids of pathogenic organisms causing disruption and eventually death.

Bacteria found in effluent (sewage), especially coliforms and pathogens like Salmonella, show significant sensitivity to the presence of oxygen in concentrations higher than 4 p.p.m (parts per million). Other bacteria that react to oxygen's disinfecting properties include Streptococci, Shigella, Legionella pneumophila, Pseudomonas aeruginosa, Yersinia enterocolitica, Campylobacter jejuni, Mycobacteria, Kiebsiella pneumonia, and Escherichia coli.

Protozoan organisms are also disrupted by the presence of high levels of oxygen. These include Giardia, Cryptosporidium and the free-living amoebas including Acanthamoeba, Hartmonella, and Negleria. The exact anti-microbial mechanism of oxygen on these protozoans is yet unknown. Perhaps there exists a direct relationship be-

---

[19] Mammals, including humans, are made up of very small cells called mammalian cells or "eukaryotes". These differ from plant cells because they do not posses cellular walls. Eukaryotes have a defined organizational structure within the cells. In other words, eukaryotes have nucleus and organelles while bacteria do not.

tween oxidative stress, oxygen perfusion into the cytoplasm and the inactivation of metabolic functions that result in organism death.

Fungi families are also inhibited and destroyed by an exposure to oxygen. These include Candida, Aspergillus, Histoplasma, Actinomycoses, and Cryptococcus. The cell walls of fungi are multilayered and are composed of approximately 80% carbohydrates and 10% of proteins and glycoproteins. The cell walls of these organisms contain disulfide bonds. It is likely that these bonds mark the site for this oxidative inactivation. In all likelihood, however, oxygen does have the capacity to diffuse through the fungal walls into the organismic cytoplasm, thus disrupting cellular organelles and killing the organism.

A parasite is an organism that lives off its host and lives a parallel life inside our bodies, feeding off our own cells or the food we eat. Pinworm eggs can be transferred to the mouth by fingers, clothing and bedding. Blood flukes and eggs enter the body through drinking water. Trichina worm larvae enter the body from undercooked meat. Hookworms can lay up to 10,000 eggs every day in the digestive tract and can survive for up to 15 years. The tapeworm can grow to more than 33 feet in length, can lay as many as 1,000,000 eggs a day and can have as many as 4,000 segments.

Recent research estimates that 85% of the individuals living in North American have at least one form of parasite infection at any one time. Frequent symptoms of these intestinal parasite infections include irritable bowel syndrome, diarrhea and chronic fatigue syndrome.

Most parasites, especially when they are in their adult stages in the human body, are extremely sensitive to the presence of oxygen.

Chapter 4:
How do cells create their energy?

Cancer cells originate from normal body cells in two phases. The first phase is the irreversible injuring of respiration. Just as there are many remote causes of plague -- heat, insects, rats -- but only one common cause, the plague bacillus, there are a great many remote causes of cancer -- tar, rays, arsenic, pressure, urethane -- but there is only one common cause into which all other causes of cancer merge, the irreversible injuring of respiration.
Dr. Otto Warburg, M.D.
The Origin of Cancer Cells: Science (1956)

    Dr. Otto Warburg[20] is still recognized as one of the premier experts on cellular metabolism and how and why healthy cells need oxygen to create the "energy" for all life processes. Dr. Warburg went to great lengths to explain that healthy cells in the body break down the carbohydrates we eat into simple "glucose" sugars. The glucose is then stored in the cells. The cells, when they need energy to perform their functions, (reproduction, heat, etc.,) take the stored glucose and, in a chemical reaction with oxygen, create A.T.P. (adenosine triphosphate) which becomes, as described by Dr. Warburg, the "pure energy of the cell."[21] If there is a lack of oxygen at the cellular level, no life processes can take place and the cell dies.

---

[20] Dr. Warburg received a Nobel Peace Prize for Medicine based on his research findings on the importance of oxygen to cellular life in 1931 and a second Nobel Prize in 1944 for his discovery of the hydrogen transferring enzymes! He was, until his retirement, the Director of the Max Planck Institute for Cell Physiology in Berlin, Germany. The complete text of his lecture delivered before the German Central Committee for Cancer Control in Stuttgart in 1955, and quoted in Science, is in Appendix VII. It is invaluable information on cellular oxygen metabolism.

[21] Warburg, O., 1969, The Prime Cause and Prevention of Cancer, (1966 Lindau Lecture, English Edition by D. Burke), Wurzburg, Germany: K. Trilsch.

But Dr. Warburg also discovered that a poor supply of oxygen is also detrimental to the cell. When cells lack the right amount of oxygen, the glucose in these cells begins to ferment and a chain reaction takes place. Instead of living off the A.T.P., the cell begins to live off of the fermentation of the stored glucose. This reverses the cell's normal metabolic cycle.

The by-products of this fermentation process produce additional toxins which leak out into the blood stream causing additional cellular damage and the suppression of the immune system. The damaged cells begin to multiply, no longer functioning as they were designed to assist the body in its various metabolic functions. These unhealthy cells (malignant or benign) drain the body of its nutritional supplies and grow in a rapid and unchecked fashion. We call groups of these cells "tumors" and the cells themselves are called "cancerous".

Here is what Dr. Warburg said in a lecture delivered in 1966 in Lindau Germany to a peer group of distinguished Nobel science recipients:

> *"Summarized in a few words, the prime cause of cancer is the replacement of the respiration of oxygen in normal cells by a fermentation of sugar. All normal body cells meet their energy needs by respiration of oxygen, whereas cancer cells meet their energy needs in great part by fermentation. All normal cells are thus obligate aerobes, whereas all cancer cells are partial anaerobes. From the standpoint of physics and the chemistry of life, this difference between normal and cancer cells is so great that one can scarcely picture a greater difference. Oxygen gas, the donor of energy in plants and animals, is dethroned in the cancer cells and replaced by an energy yielding reaction of the lowest living forms, namely, a fermentation of glucose. As emphasized, it is the first precondition of*

the proposed treatment that all growing bodies be saturated with oxygen." [22]

The research by Dr. Warburg emphasizes the important point that without an adequate supply of oxygen, the body cannot function properly. Oxygen is absolutely the most important elemental nutritional substance the body can possess. An abundant and consistent supply of oxygen is the basis for a healthy immune system and all bodily functions.

Thus, the lack of a consistent and quality supply of oxygen is considered by many medical experts as the root cause of all diseases that attack and destroy the body. Reduce the oxygen supply and we inhibit the production of energy, energy needed to maintain growth and the health of the body, energy needed to reduce or eliminate toxins in the body.

Research Studies:
Oxygen Kills Cancer Cells

A new study, completed by researchers at the University of Washington (Seattle), supports the conclusions made by Dr. Warburg more than 50 years ago: cancer cannot thrive in an oxygen-rich environment.

"An environment of pure oxygen at three-and-a-half times normal air pressure adds significantly to the effectiveness of a natural compound already shown to kill cancerous cells, researchers at the University of Washington and Washington State University recently reported in the journal Anticancer Re-

---

[22] The complete text of his presentation is in Appendix Three.

search...In the new study, using artemisinin[23], or high-pressure oxygen alone, on a culture of human leukemia cells, reduced the cancer cells' growth by 15 percent. Using them in combination reduced the cells' growth by 38 percent, a 50 percent increase in artemisinin's effectiveness."[24]

How Cells Harvest Energy

There are two ways that cells can harvest energy from food: fermentation and cellular respiration. Both start with the same first step: the process of glycolysis. Glycolysis is the breakdown (or the splitting) of a glucose molecule (containing 6 carbon atoms) into two 3-carbon molecules each called pyruvic acid. The energy derived from other sugars, like fructose, is also harvested using this same process.

Glycolysis is probably the oldest known way of producing ATP, the cell's energy source. There is evidence that the process of glycolysis predates the existence of oxygen (O_2) in the Earth's atmosphere and organelles in cells. Glycolysis occurs in the cytoplasm of cells, not in some specialized organelle, and is the singular metabolic energy pathway found in all living organisms.

---

[23] In the the 1970s, a research team, on an archeological dig in China, discovered a medicinal recipe dating back to 163 B.C. The formula featured an extract from a leafy herb called wormwood that the Chinese used to cure malaria, hemorrhoids and parasitic infections. In subsequent tests, scientists discovered that the extract, which they called "artemisinin", possessed remarkable anti-inflammatory and anti-parasitic properties. They also found that artemisinin cured malaria and that, in combination with iron, it destroyed cancer cells. Artemisinin works by releasing free radicals when exposed to oxygen. The free radicals attack and kill cancer's iron-rich cells. The killing effect can be amplified by sending additional iron to cancer cells.

[24] Hickey, Hannah. "High dose of oxygen enhances natural cancer treatment", WEB: April 4, 2011
http://www.washington.edu/news/articles/high-dose-of-oxygen-enhances-natural-cancer-treatment

Cellular Respiration:

An analogy can be drawn between the process of cellular respiration in our cells and a car's engine. The mitochondria are the engines of our cells, where sugar is burned for fuel and the exhaust is CO_2 and H_2O (water). Coincidentally, in a car that burns fuel perfectly, the only exhaust is CO_2 and H_2O, just like the end products of cellular respiration.

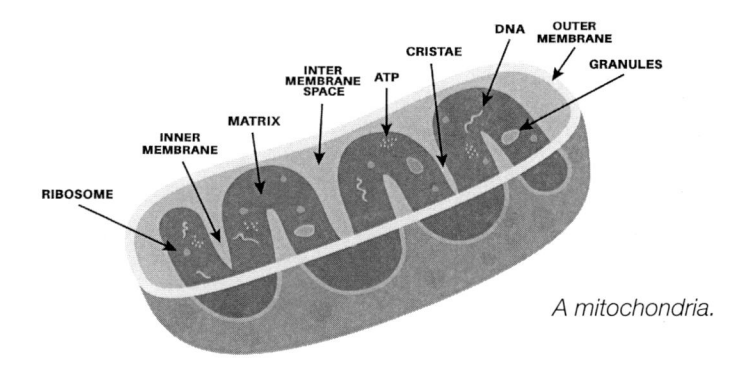

A mitochondria.

Mitochondria are the cell's equivalent of a power station. A power station burns fuel to build up steam pressure and uses that pressure to drive a turbine linked to a dynamo. This in turn generates electricity. In mitochondria, the fuel is oxidized and builds up the pressure of hydrogen ions (H^+ protons). These protons force themselves through molecular turbines and enable the cell to generate ATP (adenosine triphosphate), the energy unit that is used throughout every cell.

Just as you can work out a power station's efficiency by seeing how much electricity it produces for each unit of oxygen and fuel it burns, you can determine the efficiency of mitochondria by monitoring the amount of ATP produced for every unit of oxygen used.

For example, researchers from the University of Washington compared resting muscle cells in young (7-month) and old (30-month) mice. They found that old muscles used around half as much energy as young muscles, but that the mitochondria used just as much oxygen at both ages. This represents a 50% loss in efficiency. Author David Marcinek, The Department of Radiology, University of Washington, wrote:

> *"The best explanation for this loss of efficiency is that the mitochondria become leaky as they get old. Protons leak back into the mitochondria without making ATP, and so reduce the coupling between oxygen use and ATP production."*[25]

This inefficiency means that the muscles in older individuals produce less useable energy (ATP) for every unit of oxygen consumed. This makes normal activities seem more challenging and limiting.

There are three steps in the process of cellular respiration: glycolysis, the Krebs life cycle, and the electron transport chain. In the process of cellular respiration, pyruvic acid molecules are broken down completely to carbon dioxide (CO_2) and more energy is released. Three molecules of oxygen (as O_2) must react with each molecule of pyruvic acid to form the three carbon dioxide molecules. Three molecules of water are also formed to consume the hydrogen atoms from the original water molecules in this

---

[25] "Oxygen regulation and limitation to cellular respiration in mouse skeletal muscle in vivo",
David J. Marcinek,1 Wayne A. Ciesielski, Kevin E. Conley,1,2 and Kenneth A. Schenkman, Departments of Radiology, Physiology and Biophysics and Bioengineering, and Pediatrics, Anesthesiology, and Bioengineering, University of Washington Medical Center, Seattle, WA 98195; and Children's Hospital and Regional Medical Center, Seattle, Washington 98105. Submitted 11 March 2003. http://ajpheart.physiology.org/content/285/5/H1900.abstract

process. As mentioned above, in glycolysis, a total of four molecules of ATP are produced, but two are used up in other steps in the process.

Cellular Respiration

$$C_6H_{12}O_6 + 6O_2 \longrightarrow 6CO_2 + 6H_2O + \text{Energy}$$

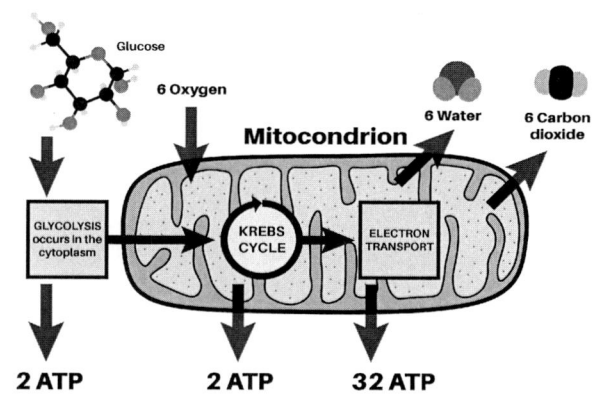

In cellular respiration, carbohydrates in the form of the simple sugar "glucose" are combined with oxygen in the cellular organelles called mitochondria. As the glucose is oxidized energy is created in the form of ATP (adenosine triphosphate) with water and carbon dioxide as waste products.

Additional ATP is produced during the Krebs Cycle and the Electron Transport Chain, resulting in a grand total of 40 ATP energy molecules produced from the breakdown of one molecule of glucose, utilizing oxygen, during cellular respiration. Since two of those ATP energy molecules are used up during glycolysis, a net total of 38 molecules of ATP are produced by cellular respiration.

In glycolysis and the Krebs cycle, there are also a number of electrons released as the glucose molecule is broken down. The cell must deal with these electrons in some way, so they are stored by the cell by forming a compound called NADH. NADH is used to carry electrons to the electron transport chain[26], where more energy is harvested.

Many of the compounds that make up the electron transport chain belong to a special group of chemicals called cytochromes. The central structure of a cytochrome is a porphyrin ring, similar to chlorophyll, but with iron in the center. (The major difference between the two rings is that chlorophyll has magnesium atom in the center of the ring.) A porphyrin with iron in the center is called a heme group, and these heme groups are also found in hemoglobin in our red blood cells used to transport oxygen.

The similarities between chlorophyl and hemoglobin molecules are uncanny. The main difference is the mineral atom at the center of each molecule. Human blood uses iron (Fe) while plant chlorophyll uses magnesium (Mg).

At the last step in the electron transport chain, the "used up" electrons, along with some "spare" hydrogen ions, are combined with O_2 to form water as a waste prod-

---

[26] The electron transport chain is a system of electron carriers embedded into the inner membranes of the mitochondria. As electrons are passed from one compound to the next in the chain, their energy is harvested and stored by forming ATP.

uct. Thus, without oxygen, the process of glycolysis and the production of energy could never take place in our cells!

A Brief Word About Cofactors and Coenzymes:

Many of the enzymes in the cells of organisms need other helpers to function properly. These non-protein enzyme helpers are called cofactors and can include substances like iron, zinc, or copper. If a cofactor is an organic molecule, it then is called a coenzyme. Many of the vitamins needed by our bodies are used as coenzymes to help our enzymes to do their jobs.

Vitamin B (thiamine) is a coenzyme used in removing waste CO_2 from various organic compounds. Vitamin B_2 (riboflavin) is a component of FAD (or $FADH_2$), one of the chemicals used to transport electrons from the Krebs cycle to the electron transport chain needed to produce ATP oxygen energy. Vitamin B_3 (niacin) is a component of NAD + (or NADH), which is the major transporter of electrons from glycolysis and the Krebs cycle to the electron transport chain which creates more energy from oxygen. Vitamin B_6 (pyridoxine), Vitamin B_{12} (cobalamin), pantothenic acid, folic acid, and biotin are other B vitamins that serve as coenzymes at various points in metabolizing our food and creating energy. Interestingly, B_{12} has a cobalt atom in it, which is a mineral that we need in only very minute quantities, but whose absence can seriously affect our ability to create cellular energy. Without enough of these B vitamins, and oxygen, our ability to get the energy out of our food would come to a grinding halt!

Chapter 5:
When the Immune System Breaks Down

Oxygen plays a pivotal role in the proper functioning of the immune system.
Dr. Parris M. Kidd, Ph.D.[27]
Antioxidant Adaptation

The immune system is a remarkable defensive mechanism that is designed to work flawlessly to defend the body against deadly invading microorganisms. Perhaps one of the best descriptions of this highly organized network was published by the National Institute of Allergy and Infectious Diseases:

> *"The immune system is a network of cells, tissues, and organs that work together to defend the body against attacks by 'foreign' invaders. These are primarily microbes—tiny organisms such as bacteria, parasites, and fungi that can cause infections. Viruses also cause infections, but are too primitive to be classified as living organisms. The human body provides an ideal environment for many microbes. It is the immune system's job to keep them out or, failing that, to seek out and destroy them...The immune system is amazingly complex. It can recognize and remember millions of different*

---

[27] Dr. Parris Kidd, PhD. earned his Bachelor of Science Degree in Zoology and Marine Biology and his PhD at the University of California, Berkeley in cell biology. He then received grants from the California Heart Association and the United States National Institutes of Health to study heart and blood vessel disease. Dr. Kidd has written books and numerous articles on antioxidants, cell membrane molecules, enzyme cofactors, and all the other dietary substances that improve health and help prevent disease.Dr. Kidd has been a contributing editor and science advisor to Total Health magazine since 1996.

enemies, and it can produce secretions (release of fluids) and cells to match up with and wipe out nearly all of them. The secret to its success is an elaborate and dynamic communications network. Millions and millions of cells, organized into sets and subsets, gather like clouds of bees swarming around a hive and pass information back and forth in response to an infection. Once immune cells receive the alarm, they become activated and begin to produce powerful chemicals. These substances allow the cells to regulate their own growth and behavior, enlist other immune cells, and direct the new recruits to trouble spots."[28]

Dr. Stephen Levine[29] and Dr. Parris M. Kidd, (both well respected molecular biologists,) conducted research that confirmed that "...oxygen is the source of life to all cells."[30] Their medical research indicated that we subject our bodies to massive amounts of physiological stress because of poor eating and drinking habits and a lack of exercise. These two factors alone rob precious oxygen from our bodies.

---

[28] "What is the Immune System?". U.S. Department of Health and Human Services, National Institute of Health
http://www.niaid.nih.gov/topics/immuneSystem/pages/whatisimmunesystem.aspx

[29] Stephen Levine, PhD, is the founder of Allergy Research Group, and heads up its Scientific Advisory Board. Dr. Levine graduated Cum Laude from the State University College, Buffalo, NY and obtained his PhD from the University of California, Berkeley in Molecular Biology. Dr. Levine was a Horace and Edith King Davis Memorial Fellow; recipient of an NIH Training Grant, and Predoctoral Fellow, 1972 - 1976. Dr. Levine is internationally recognized as one of the foremost innovative leaders and researchers in nutritional supplement formulation. He is recognized as an international lecturer with several editorial positions in professionally sought after publications. Dr. Levine also co-authored, with Parris M Kidd PhD, the book "Antioxidant Adaptation: Its Role in Free Radical Pathology," which is considered a leading resource on this subject.

[30] Levine, Dr. Stephen. Biocurrents Press. Biocurrents Research and Development, Corporation. 944 Lake Street, San Francisco, CA, (415) 639-4575.

This situation is further complicated by the presence of pollutants and toxic chemicals in the water and food we consume and the air we breathe. Research reveals that in the last 30 years, our food and water supplies in the U.S. and around the world have been contaminated by over 70,000 new toxic substances that our bodies must now try to metabolize. Each year, we produce over 100,000,000 tons of synthetic chemicals, any one of which can seriously affect the immune system and our health. Dr. Levine continues:

> *"We can look at oxygen deficiency as the single greatest cause of all diseases.."*[31]

It is believed, and supported by a great deal of research, that a shortage of oxygen in the blood could very well be the starting point for the breakdown of the immune system. According to Dr. Levine, "oxygen nutrition" optimizes the concentration of oxygen in relation to a natural food diet. In other words, the amount of oxygen in relation to food density is the key for excellent cellular metabolism. Dr. Levine went further and explained that complex carbohydrates are oxygen rich foods. These complex carbohydrates include vegetables, whole grains, seeds, and nuts. (Fruits are too high in simple sugars to be classified as complex carbohydrates.)

As a research chemist, Dr. Levine defines a complex carbohydrate as having 16 parts of oxygen and only 14 parts carbon and hydrogen.

> *"More than half the weight of complex carbohydrates is oxygen. But the percentage of oxygen in fats is less than ten or at the very most fifteen percent, so fats are very low in oxygen. In fact, fats are*

---

[31] Ibid.

oxygen robbers. Protein is composed of 0 to 50 percent oxygen, depending on the specific amino acid profile. It is obvious that complex carbohydrates have the most oxygen."[32]

No nutrient - whether it is protein, fatty acid, vitamin or mineral - fulfills its functions in its original form. Nutrients, as they occur in our diets, are simply mechanical substances necessary for converting the potential energy in our foods into usable chemical energy for living. For this conversion to take place, oxygen must be present.

Dr. Warburg's research adds further emphasis to these findings. He stated that sub-optimal oxygenation of tissues and cells as seen in cellular hypoxia, (a lack of oxygen at the cellular level,) is not only the underlying cause of diseases, like cancer, but also results in a predisposition towards degenerative diseases.

The lack of oxygen is the primary factor in immune-depressive illnesses. Thus, these researchers conclude, the increased oxygenation of the blood stream and cells will most certainly enhance, and may even restore, overall health.[33]

Oxygen is used by the cells in many processes that break down toxic substances in the body. This process of combining a substance with oxygen at the cellular level is called "oxidation". Dr. Levine describes "oxidation" this way:

"Oxygen provides the spark of life. Nutrients provide the fuel for burning. The correct fuel/oxygen mixture is required for the best of health."[34]

---

[32] op. cit. Levine and Kidd "Antioxidant Adaptation"

[33] op. cit. Warburg, The Prime Cause and Prevention of Cancer
op. cit. Warburg, The Lindau Lecture. Germany.

[34] op. cit. Levine and Kidd, "Antioxidant Adaptation"

A lack of oxygen in proper amounts prevents oxidation and oxygenation, two processes that energize the cells to biological regeneration. These processes are the very foundation of life and death. If the normal environment of the cell is maintained, it will not lose its growth and reproduction potential. Poor oxygen supplies will result in poor oxidation. Poor oxidation results in increased cellular contamination.

Oxygen is a vital cell detoxifier. When body oxygen levels are deficient, toxins build and may eventually devastate the body's metabolic functions and deplete the body of life-giving energy.

Without oxygen, there can be no nourishment. Without nourishment, there can be no heat nor energy and the body cannot purify itself. A body with an excellent oxygen supply, and an unhindered functioning of oxidation and oxygenation metabolic processes, will be healthier.

Chapter 6:
Free Radicals:
Enemies or Allies

When there is excessive oxidation and a deficiency of antioxidants, the excess free radicals are free to create havoc in the body. They are involved in aging, immune diseases, cancer and, of course, in chemical sensitivities and allergies.
Dr. Abram Hoffer, M.D., Ph.D.[35]

Minute amounts of free radicals are essential for many important functions of the immune system and other vital cellular activities.
Dr. Peter Rothschild, M.D.
Free Radicals, Stress and Antioxidant Enzymes[36]

Over the last 30 years, thousands of scientific studies have revealed that free radical activity represents a major cause of all degenerative diseases. These same studies also indicate, quite clearly, that there is an effective way to control, and in some cases eliminate, most free radical damage.

Unfortunately, free radical science is totally misunderstood by the general public. Misinformation on this subject, especially as it relates to the claim that oxygen is a dangerous substance to the body, is often promoted by both the media and by manufacturers of nutrients and dietary

---

[35] Born in Southern Saskatchewan, Canada, earned a Masters degree in agricultural chemistry in 1940. After completing a PhD in 1944, he became interested in human nutrition, earning his M.D. in 1949. He qualified in psychiatry in 1954 and became a Fellow in the Royal College of Physicians and Surgeons (Canada). Dr Hoffer and co-workers were instrumental in the discovery that megadoses of vitamin B3 (nicotinic acid/niacin) was therapeutic for schizophrenia and can be used to lower cholesterol levels. Their discovery, published in 1955, is credited with the initiation of the new paradigm in nutritional medicine, i.e. the use of vitamins for treatment and not just for prevention of deficiency disease.

[36] Dr. Peter Rothschild, Free Radicals, Stress and Antioxidant Enzymes. University Labs Press, Honolulu, Hawaii. 1991; 3-4.

health supplements. What is the truth? What actually is a free radical? How and why are they created? Are all free radicals harmful to the body? Is there an effective way to deactivate or control free radicals? Finally, is oxygen the real villain that it has been made out to be and is oxygen responsible for producing free radicals?

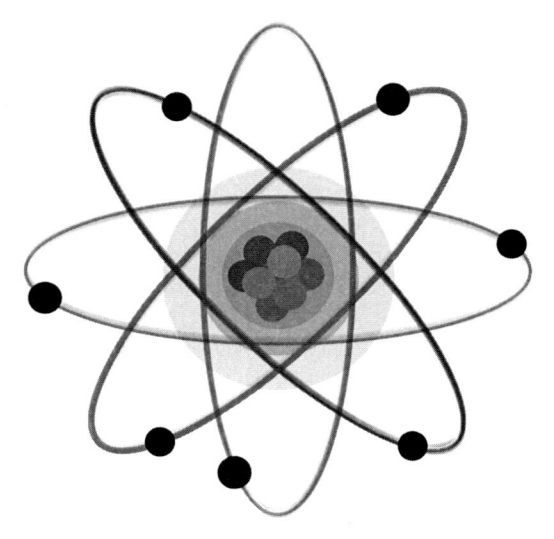

A free radical atom is missing an electron in its outermost shell (valence).

Before we take a more in-depth look into how free radicals "react" in the body, let's look at how the experts describe these unusual atoms molecules. Dr. Denham Harman, M.D., Ph.D. is considered the "father" of free radical aging theory. A professor emeritus at the University of Nebraska, Omaha, Dr. Harman put forth the belief back in 1954 that unstable atoms called "free radicals" cause damage to cellular DNA that result in cellular death. Thus, free radicals, he believed, were the cause of the aging process.

"Chances are that 99% are the basis for aging. Aging is the ever increasing accumulation of changes caused or contributed to by free radicals."[37]

Dr. Earl Stadtman, M.D., Chief of the Laboratory of Biochemistry of the National Heart, Lung and Blood Institute in Bethesda, M.D. concurs with Dr. Harman:

"What the human life span reflects is simply the level of free radical oxidative damage that accumulates in the cells. When enough damage accumulates, cells can't survive properly anymore and they just give up."[38]

The simplest definition of a free radical was written by Dr. Kurt Donsbach, N.D. in his book Oxygen-Oxygen-Oxygen:

"It is an element or compound which has an unpaired or unmatched electron. This lack of balance causes the substance to have a very reactive character. However, it must be noted that these free radicals are very short-lived, usually in the one ten-thousandth of a second range. But during this short time, these free radicals can cause damage by joining with other body chemicals and changing their character, sometimes even producing a chain reaction by creating new free radicals that carry on."[39]

---

[37] Challem, Jack. "Free Radicals and Antioxidants: A Contrarian View?" Nutrition Review, Natural Food Merchandiser Nutrition Science News, December 1995.

Corner, Peter and Ronald Kotulak. "Scientists Try to Tame Molecular 'Sharks.'" Chicago Tribune, December 11, 1991.

[38] Ibid. Corner.

[39] Donsbach, Kurt, N.D., Ph.D. Oxygen - Oxygen - Oxygen Rockland Corporation: 1993; 13.

Dr. Peter Rothschild, M.D., in his work Free Radicals, Stress and Antioxidant Enzymes wrote:

> *"Due to their over-reactive nature, free radicals can be extremely toxic and are a direct consequence of the primary stress factors that adversely affect the immune system and threaten our health. However, this is not to imply that free radicals are always harmful or dangerous. Minute amounts of free radicals are essential for many important functions of the immune system and other vital cellular activities. For example, the immune system will actually generate free radicals to use in the process of removing a virus or bacteria. Only when high concentrations of free radicals are present, or when the levels of free radicals overwhelm the body's ability to remove them, does a threat to our health occur. Maintaining the balance between free radical activity and antioxidant enzyme supply is one of the important functions of the body."*[40]

Free radicals are missing electrons, and in this quantum atomic state, they will do whatever they can in grabbing an electron from another source. Around every atom orbits electrons in what are called shells. These shells (or sub-orbits) vary in distance from the center of the atom's nucleus.

Each sub-orbit can accommodate two electrons, each "spinning" in a different direction, and generating what quantum physicists call "wave forms" or "wave packets". If one of these electrons is missing in the outer orbit, the atom will seek out a matching electron. The atom will not stop looking for this match until it finds one. Such an unstable and reactive atom is called a free radical.

---

[40] Rothshild, Peter R. and Fahey, William. Free Radicals, Stress and Antioxidant Enzymes. University Labs Press, Honolulu, HI: 1991; 3-4.

Stable Molecule   **Unstable Molecule**
(Free Radical)

A stable oxygen atom (left) has a balanced number of rotating electrons (8) around its nucleus. An unstable atom (right), called a "free radical", is missing a rotating electron. In this state it must find an electron from another atom or molecule in order to reach a stable state.

Free radicals can be various sizes, from single atoms to more complex molecules. They can be one, two, three and four atom molecules based on oxygen, or may be formed combining with other atoms. The most destructive free radial molecules include superoxide, hydrogen peroxide, hydroxyl, singlet oxygen (not diatomic oxygen or O_2), polyunsaturated fatty acids, organic/fatty acid hydroperoxides and oxidized proteins.[41]

It is important to point out that oxygen is not the "cause" of free radical production in the body. In fact, oxygen does not cause free radicals any more than glucose causes energy production. It is true that if the body did not contain oxygen, then no oxygen free radicals could be created. This seems like a paradox, and in some ways it is. The body produces oxygen free radicals as a natural part of metabolic energy production in every cell. As oxygen is consumed, along with glucose, to produce A.T.P. energy, some of the by-products of metabolism are oxygen free-radicals.

The body needs energy to carry out daily functions, like cellular growth, cellular replacement, maintaining body temperature, muscle actions (movement) and thinking. All of these processes require enormous amounts of energy.

---

[41] Challem, Jack. "Free Radicals and Antioxidants: A Contrarian View?" Nutrition Review, Natural Food Merchandiser Nutrition Science News, December 1995.

Again, this energy is derived from the combustion of oxygen and glucose in power plants in each cell called the mitochondria. Like a factory that burns fuel for energy and produces smoke, the mitochondria produce waste products that we call free radicals.

Free Radicals:
Superoxide (O_2^-)
Hydrogen Peroxide (H_2O_2)
Hydroxyl Radical (OH^-)
Singlet Oxygen ($^-O_2$)
Hydroperoxy Radical (HOO^-)
Lipid Peroxide Radical (ROO^-)
Nitric Oxide (NO^-)
Peroxynitrite ($ONOO^-$)
Chlorine (Cl^-)

Different types of free radicals. Not all free radicals contain oxygen atoms.

There are, of course, sources of free radicals other than those produced in the mitochondria during the combustion of oxygen and glucose. The free radicals from these sources may react with oxygen free radicals to create different molecules that can cause even more damage. The sources for these destructive free radicals include alcohol, tobacco smoke, nicotine, industrial pollution and other emissions, pesticides, pollution in water, food and the air, saturated and overheated fats, smog, radiation (including ultraviolet/ U.V.), organic solvents, unprotected exposure to sunlight, detergents, paints, cleaning solvents, hair sprays, deodorants and more. It is the accumulation of these toxins that cause the greatest damage to the human body. And these pollutants rob oxygen from the body.

Now, if the body produces free radicals as it generates energy, it only stands to reason that the body must have some mechanism to control these oxygen free radicals as they are continuously created. If the body did not have such protection, and if, as the theory states, that oxygen free radicals can cause cellular D.N.A. damage, then without such protection the body would soon deteriorate and die. So, how does the body protect itself?

The body protects itself by utilizing the electrochemical uniqueness of antioxidants. Antioxidants are a group of atoms and molecules that bond with or share electrons with free radicals making these radicals stable atoms or molecules. This means that free radicals can be controlled by molecules and atoms produced in the body, like the enzymes superoxide dismutase (SOD) and glutathione peroxidase, as well as naturally occurring vitamins and nutrients we can consume from foods, like E, C, beta-carotene and bioflavonoids. These free radical soldiers or "scavengers" deactivate free radicals.

Superoxide dismutase, produced by the body, is perhaps the most important defender against free radicals. In fact it is so important that out of over 100,000 proteins that the body produces, it is the fifth most prevalent. SOD is powerful in its ability to eliminate superoxide (O_2-) molecules.[42]

As mentioned earlier, there are both good and bad free radicals. As Joanne McAllister Smart, Managing Editor of Vegetarian Times, writes:

> *"Free radicals are not all bad -- at least not if you count breathing among life's more positive experiences. Ironically, breathing is the major source of free radical production in humans. Because oxygen molecules have not one, but two unpaired electrons, the most common free radicals are built on oxygen. All living things require energy to function. As humans we need a lot of energy to think, eat,*

---

[42] Cichoke, Dr. Anthony, M.A., D.C., D.A.C.B.N., "Inside / Out." The Energy Times, July / August 1994.

sleep, talk and other fun things. To generate energy, cells remove electrons from sugars and add these electrons to oxygen forming highly reactive compounds. Most of these temporarily unstable molecules eventually combine with hydrogen to form stable water molecules...Free radicals are also purposely created by the immune system to fight against invading bacteria and viruses."[43]

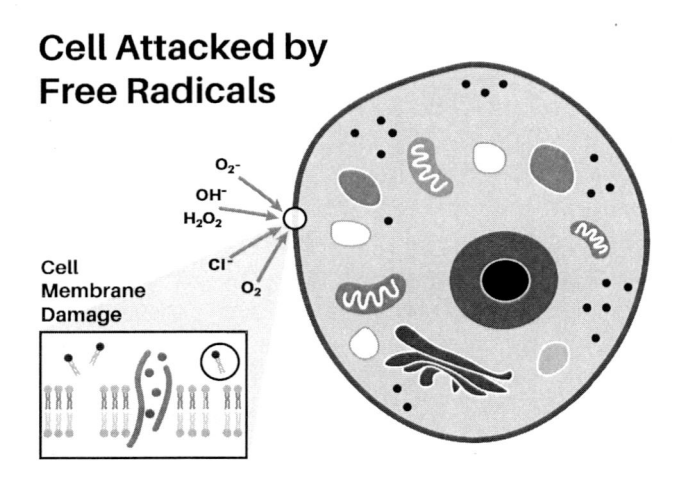

Cell Attacked by Free Radicals

O_2^-
OH^-
H_2O_2
Cl^-
O_2

Cell Membrane Damage

When a cell comes into contact with a free radical there is a rapid exchange of electrons from the host cell to the free radical. When this occurs, the cellular membrane disintegrates (see box at left). This causes a breach in the cell's integrity. Soon after this rupture occurs, the cell's contents leak out and the cell either becomes damaged or dies..

The body produces free radicals as an important component of the immune system. But free radicals are supposed to cause aging, sickness and death! Do we have another paradox to deal with? Yes.

---

[43] McAllister Smart. "Antioxidants for the Uninitiated." Vegetarian Times, April 1994.

I started out this chapter stating that oxygen is a double-edged sword. Without oxygen we die. With oxygen we subject ourselves to free-radicals as the body naturally produces energy to function and live. With oxygen we also produce the first line of defense used by our immune system in its daily battle against an invading army of pathogens that includes viruses, bacteria, yeasts and molds. Jack Challem, a featured writer to a number of health related publications, and editor of the Nutrition Reporter, a publication that summarizes recent medical journal articles on vitamins and nutrition, explains this relationship between "the good, the bad and the ugly" this way:

> *"It's necessary to know that free radicals, while often the villains in what has popularly been branded as a 'biological gunfight at the OK Corral' are not always the bad guys. Free radicals are sometimes the good guys. For example, white blood cells use free radicals to destroy bacteria and virus-infected cells. According to Bruce Ames, Ph.D., of the University of California, Berkeley, these free radicals prevent immediate death from infection. In addition, with the help of other free radicals, the liver's cytochrome P-450 enzymes detoxify harmful chemicals. What contributes to disease and rapid aging are excessive free radicals produced by outside environmental influences. If you wipe out large numbers of good free radicals, you're handcuffing your body's immune system."*[44]

Mr. Challem delves deeper into the free radical controversy in a subsequent article he wrote for Nutrition Science News. He explained that the body produces free radicals in four ways. First, most are produced as a consequence of eating and breathing. As the body produces

---

[44] Challem, Jack. "Are You Overdoing Antioxidants?" Natural Health, May/June 1995.

energy some superoxide free radicals escape and can cause cellular DNA damage. (By the way, anything that increases respiration, including exercise, also increases free radical production!)

Second, as fatty acids are digested or broken down, hydrogen peroxide molecules (H_2O_2) are created. Some of these peroxide molecules escape and can oxidize fats in the membranes of cells thus damaging the permeability and the integrity of the membranes.

Third, enzymes produced in the liver, (like cytochrome P450,) are designed to detoxify the body from pollutants contained in water, food, air, smoke as well as other chemicals or toxins occurring naturally in foods. P450 thus helps prevent acute illnesses and rapid death from these poisons to our bodies. But, as P450 and other enzymes break down these toxins, free radicals are produced that can injure healthy tissues and contribute to aging and death.

Fourth, white blood cells, the body's foot soldiers against invading diseases, produce tremendous amounts of free radicals to fight infections. White blood cells "digest" bacteria and virus-infected cells and kill these pathogenic organisms with a shotgun-like burst of free radicals (hydroxyl, superoxide, peroxide and singlet oxygen.) These same bullets can also hit and damage healthy cells.[45]

Dr. Howard Halperin, M.D. at the University of Chicago adds a fifth way the body produces beneficial free radicals. He writes:

> *"One of life's most beautiful and dramatic moments occurs when a newborn infant takes its first breath. A baby's ability to switch quickly from its mother's circulation and take oxygen into its lungs is generated by a type of free radical."*[46]

---

[45] op. cit. Challem "Free Radicals and Antioxidants"

[46] Corner, Peter and Ronald Kotulak. "Scientists Try to Tame Molecular 'Sharks.'" Chicago Tribune, December 11, 1991.

Dr. Robert Koch, discoverer of the tubercle bacillus (the cause of tuberculosis), and a staunch supporter of oxygen-based therapies, explained the purpose of free radicals in the immune system in more scientific terms:

> "When its (oxygen's) activity wanes, the toxins that support pathogenic germ activity, that produce allergy, or that cause cancer, are not destroyed in the body and can execute their effects. All of these toxins depend upon their free valences between carbon atoms, between carbon and oxygen, and between carbon and nitrogen for their pathogenic action. Our synthetic antitoxins not only activate oxygen, but they activate the toxic free valences of germ and allergy poisons to accept the activated oxygen and thus become burned to harmless structures."[47]

Without a doubt, free radicals can do damage to the cells in our body. Recent studies indicate that free radicals bombard cellular DNA molecules over 10,000 time a day but severe cellular injury seldom occurs because of the body's natural antioxidant defense mechanisms.[48] In fact, according to research conducted by Dr. Bruce Ames, Director of the National Institute of Environmental Health Sciences Center at the University of California in Berkeley, these naturally produced antioxidant enzymes, vitamins, minerals and proteins race to these accident scenes and repair the damage from 99% to 99.9% of the time![49]

---

[47] Morales, Betty Lee. 'The Free Radical- The Common Denominator of Disease." Let's Live, July 1982.

[48] op. cit. Corner and Kotulak. "Scientists Try to Tame Molecular 'Sharks.'"

Walker, Dr. Morton, D.P.M. "Fruit & Vegetable Antioxidants: New Research." Health Food Business, July 1995.

[49] Ibid. Corner.

Dr. Ames' research goes on the explain that the real problem is that the body simply cannot keep up with this constant repair cycle and so the result is aging. Thus, as Dr. Ames points out, the life spans of animals and humans are directly related the the body's ability to repair free radical damage. He writes:

> "Normally we're OK. But it doesn't quite keep up. As you get older, more and more ... accumulates. Sunshine, for instance, is a carcinogen and 99% of its damage is repaired. But if you get too much sunshine, you get skin cancer and melanoma."[50]

Dr. Earl Stadtman, M.D. adds:

> "What the human life span reflects is simply the level of oxidative damage that accumulates in the cells...When enough damage accumulates, cells can't survive properly anymore and they just give up."[51]

It's important to mention one more time that free radicals are not left to do damage without a very efficient safety net in our bodies. This net includes the actions and reactions of groups of powerful free radical scavengers that neutralize these radicals and prevent massive cell oxidation. They accomplish this by either supplying the missing electron to a free radical or removing an electron which stabilizes the free radical and thus stops its potential danger.

Finally, some exceptional research completed in 2012 at the University of California at Davis and the National Children's Research Center (Ireland) discovered that reactive oxygen species (ROS) are not what actually kills

---

[50] Ibid.

[51] Ibid.

pathogens, as was believed for many decades. Instead, as the researchers discovered,

> "...ROS interfere with the signaling process needed to produce the protective capsule around Campylobacter bacteria. Without this capsule, the bacteria are less capable of causing and sustaining infection."[52]

Therefore, free radicals are actually the first line of defense against bacterial infections.

Since we know where free radicals come from and how they are created, does science also know how to reduce their effects on the body? An increasingly broad spectrum of research indicates we do indeed have part of the solution. Though we cannot stop breathing, which is the source of oxygen to keep us alive, but is also a source (not the cause!) of free radicals, we can prevent the build-up of toxins and pollutants which cause the most dangerous group of free radicals that are in the air we breathe, water we drink and food we consume.

We can also assist the body in fighting off the aging process by making sure we have a sufficient supply of antioxidant missiles in our defensive arsenal against disease. High quality and bio-available vitamin, mineral and amino acid supplements are available from numerous companies. Fresh fruits, herbs and vegetables also supply very potent antioxidants to the body.

Free radicals are an instrumental part of the body's working mechanisms. Oxygen free radicals serve an important and critical cleansing and disinfecting purpose. Without them, sick cells, toxins and disease organisms could not

---

[52] Corcionivoschi et al (2012) Mucosal Reactive Oxygen Species Decrease Virulence by Disrupting Campylobacter jejuni Phosphotyrosine Signaling. Cell Host & Microbe 12, 47–59, July 19, 2012 dx.doi.org/10.1016. 2012.05.018

be controlled or eliminated. Author and nutritionist Sonya Starr writes:

> "Without the free radical oxygen, also known as O_1 or nascent oxygen, 'nasty and destructive' free radicals cannot be efficiently eliminated by the body. The nascent available free radical oxygen seeks out and combines with toxic free radicals. These destructive free radicals have accumulated due to the absence of healthy 'free radical' oxygen. This absence has hindered the whole oxidative cycle of our aerobic bodies."[53]

Maharishi Ayur-Ved summarized the free radical issue in his book Freedom from Disease: How to Control Free Radicals:

> "They are an inescapable feature of all oxygen based life. As part of the life-giving process that creates energy in every cell, free radicals are created as toxic waste. When the immune systems sends special forces to fight infection, free radicals are used as a weapon...If the body takes in pesticides, industrial chemicals, processed foods, cigarette smoke, or alcohol, free radicals are the most common result. And when the mind and body come under stress, free radicals are mass produced."[54]

Lastly, many researchers would have us believe that less oxygen in the body would result in less free radical production. Therefore, they would further clarify, taking oxygen supplementation would be actually harmful to the body

---

[53] Starr, Sonya C., B.S., N.C. "Oxygen - 02: The Life Giving Element." The Nutrition & Dietary Consultant, August 1986.

[54] Ayur-Ved, Maharishi. Freedom from Disease: How to Control Free Radicals. Veda Publishing, Toronto, Canada: 1993.

since any increase in oxygen would result in a corresponding increase in free radical production. But some logical assumptions are not necessarily true.

Research conducted for the U.S. Army's Environmental Medicine Research Institute by Dr. Wayne Askew, Ph.D., now the Director of the Division of Foods and Nutrition at the University of Utah, indicates a different oxygen story. Studying oxidative stress, and the need for antioxidants at high altitudes, Dr. Askew determined that less oxygen increased oxidative stress and the need for additional antioxidant supplementation to deal with that stress.[55] To put it in another way, less oxygen to the body increases the production of free radicals as well as our need for a greater supply of antioxidants to neutralize the free radicals. Dr. Askew's findings agree with the theories proposed by Dr. Robert Koch some 60 years earlier:

> *"When adequate molecular oxygen is available, protection against disease is provided. When molecular oxygen is not available, the free radicals formed by the dehydrogenation cannot combine with oxygen and forms a peroxide-free radical to continue the combustion process. The free radical can do only one thing: add to the closest double bond at hand. This is the same double bond that activates the carbonyl group which removed its hydrogen atom to form the free radical. By this action, the host cell's energy production mechanism is paralyzed by the integration of the foreign substance of fuel product. Normal function is blocked and can be forced beyond physiological control*

---

[55] Askew, Dr. Eldon W., Ph.D. "Environmental and Physical Stress and Nutrient Requirements." American Journal of Clinical Nutrition, 1995; 61 (Suppl.): 631S-7S. American Society for Clinical Nutrition.

by the input of vicarious energy, which can result in multiple allergies and/or cancer."[56]

About Free Radicals and Aging:

Again, the conventional wisdom has held for many decades that free radicals cause aging, and that antioxidants, which squelch the reactivity of these highly reactive molecules, are a way to slow the process. But brand new research adds to a growing body of prior research that suggests the story is not so simple.

In a study published in PLoS Biology[57], worms that made more free radicals, or that were treated with a free-radical-producing herbicide, actually lived longer than normal worms. What's more, when the longer-lived mutant worms were given antioxidants, the effects were reversed, and the worms had a conventional worm lifespan. The finding flies in the face of the idea that antioxidants battle the effects of aging.

According to the study's author Siegfried Hekimi (McGill University in Montreal, Canada) and others, what is emerging from this and other experiments is a view of free radicals -- or, more precisely, reactive oxygen species -- as a normal part of the body's stress response, with beneficial effects at certain levels.

Dr. Barry Halliwell of the National University of Singapore, one of the leading researchers of reactive oxygen species stated:

---

[56] Morales, Betty Lee. 'The Free Radical- The Common Denominator of Disease." Let's Live, July 1982.

[57] Wen Yang, Siegfried Hekimi. A Mitochondrial Superoxide Signal Triggers Increased Longevity in Caenorhabditis elegans. PLoS Biology, 2010; 8 (12): e1000556 DOI: 10.1371/journal.pbio.1000556 as reported in Science News, ScienceDaily.com. "Free Radicals Good for You? Banned Herbicide Makes Worms Live Longer", Dec. 20, 2010
http://www.sciencedaily.com/releases/2010/12/101220084442.htm

> "You cannot live without them, nor should you wish to, but they will probably help to kill you in the end...Learning how to stop the latter whilst preserving the useful functions of reactive oxygen species should be a major research priority in the next few years."[58]

The bottom line: Free radicals are an important part of our body's normal functioning and may even be good for us in certain doses. Worms that made extra free radicals lived longer than typical worms, but the effect was reversed when they were treated with antioxidants. Research does not support taking more antioxidants than we consume via diet. Nor, on the other hand, is increasing oxygen consumption going to cause a rise in free radicals that can do harm to the body.

---

[58] Ibid.

Chapter 7:
Oxygen and Muscle Basics

> Insufficient oxygen means insufficient biological energy that can result in anything from mild fatigue to life threatening disease. The link between insufficient oxygen and disease has now been firmly established.
> Dr. Spencer Way, M.D.
> Journal of the American Association of Physicians

> Muscles do not use oxygen at a constant rate.
> Dr. August Krogh, Ph.D.[59]

When we exercise or play sports, we probably notice several things about our bodies: we breathe heavier and more quickly; our hearts beats faster; our muscles feel "tired" and we sweat. These are all normal responses to physical exercise whether we only have the endurance for a weekend pick-up game or are a trained athlete.

Any type of exercise uses muscles. Running, swimming, weightlifting, any sport we can imagine, uses different muscle groups to generate motion. In running and swimming, our muscles are working to accelerate our body and to keep it moving. In weightlifting, our muscles are working to move a weight. Exercise means muscle activity.

As we use our muscles, they begin to place demands on the rest of the body. During strenuous exercise, nearly every system in our body focuses its efforts on helping the muscles do their work. For example, the heart beats faster so that it can pump more blood to the muscles. The stomach shuts down so that the body does not waste the energy that the muscles need.

---

[59] August Steenberg Krogh, Ph.D. (1874-1949)was a Danish physiologist who received the Nobel Prize for Physiology in Medicine in 1920 for his discovery of the motor-regulating mechanism of capillaries (small blood vessels).

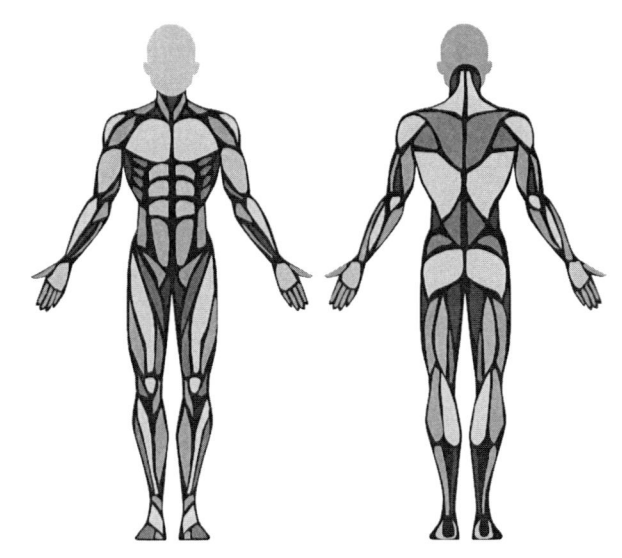

The muscles must have a dependable and continuous supply of oxygen to minimize pain, enhance muscle repair and improve stamina and endurance.

When exercising, the muscles act like electric motors. They take in a source of energy and they use it to generate force. An electric motor uses electricity to supply its energy. Muscles are biochemical motors and use ATP for their energy source. During the process of "burning" this ATP as fuel, the muscles require three things: they need oxygen, because it's needed to produce ATP; they must get rid of metabolic wastes, (like carbon dioxide, lactic acid,); they need to get rid of heat, because working muscles generate a lot of heat.

In order to continue functioning, muscles must continuously make ATP. To allow this happen, the body must supply oxygen to the muscles and remove waste products and heat. The more strenuous the activity, the greater the needs are of the working muscles. And if these needs are not met, then exhaustion sets in and the muscles fail. To meet these three needs, the body has an incredibly detailed plan involving the heart, blood vessels, nervous system, lungs and even the skin.

Oxygen for Energy

After less than two minutes of exercise, the body automatically responds by supplying the working muscles with oxygen. During physical activity, the blood vessels in the muscles dilate so that more blood can flow through these vessels and capillaries. It is like the difference between water flowing through a fire hose compared to a garden hose. Obviously, more water can flow through the fire hose because it is larger in diameter.

The blood carries the much-needed oxygen to the muscles. Blood that would have gone to the stomach or the kidneys now goes instead to the muscles. The lungs and the rest of the respiratory system now have to provide more oxygen for all the blood that is now being directed to the working muscles. That is why, when we exercise, breathing becomes more rapid and deeper. This is because sympathetic nerves stimulate the respiratory muscles to tell them to increase the number of breaths per minute.

Byproducts from muscle contractions, like carbon dioxide and lactic acid, send signals to the respiratory center in the brain, which, in turn, stimulates the respiratory muscles, telling them to work harder. Blood pressure increases, caused by the increased force of each heartbeat, and opens blood flow to more air sacs in the lungs. This permits more oxygen to enter the blood.

Now that the body has increased the flow of oxygen-rich blood to the muscles, the muscles still need to get this oxygen out of the blood. An exchange of oxygen and carbon dioxide now takes place. The iron-rich protein hemoglobin in every red blood cell, handles this task. As explained in an earlier chapter, hemoglobin binds either to oxygen or carbon dioxide.

Hemoglobin, in red blood cells that enter the lungs, has carbon dioxide bound to each heme molecule. In the lungs, the oxygen concentration is high and the carbon dioxide concentration is low. Hemoglobin grabs oxygen molecules and releases carbon dioxide molecules. The red blood cells, now saturated with oxygen, are transported through the heart, blood vessels and capillaries to the muscles. In the muscles, the carbon dioxide concentration is high and the oxygen concentration is low. Hemoglobin releases oxygen and grabs the carbon dioxide metabolic waste gas. The red blood cells are then transported back to the lungs and the cycle repeats itself.

Contracting muscles during physical activity use energy and produce wastes, like lactic acid and carbon dioxide. Acids reduce the attraction between oxygen and hemoglobin and causes the hemoglobin to release more oxygen than usual. This increases the oxygen delivered to the muscle.

To continue to function efficiently, the muscles have to dispose of their metabolic wastes. All the extra blood that flows to the muscles during increased activity also bring more oxygen. So the blood takes away the wastes.

Inside the Muscle Cell

Inside every muscle cell is the cell's "cytoplasm". (In a muscle cell the cytoplasm is called the "sarcoplasm".) This is literally everything inside of the plasma or cell membrane (sarcolemma) aside from the cell's nucleus.

The contents of a muscle cell can be broken down into two distinct areas. if you could look into a muscle fiber, it looks like it is stuffed with little threads. These threads are called "myofibrils". Myofibrils can become larger when the muscle is regularly exercised and they contain the components that allow our muscles to contract. What surrounds these tiny myofibril threads is a transparent moist gel-like substance called "Cytosol ".

A muscle allows nutrients to pass through the muscle cell's permeable membrane from the blood stream. It then stores or converts those nutrients into useable energy. So the cytosol contains amino acids, for maintenance and repair, and glycogen, a complex carbohydrate for energy.

A muscle fiber must have a fuel source in order to contract. This is why the cytosol also has tiny organs called organelles, or microscopic organs. Perhaps the most significant of these are the mitochondria. As we have learned, the mitochondria convert carbohydrates and oxygen into ATP, which is the muscle cell's main energy currency (fuel).

The macronutrient (food) stores in the sarcoplasm of every muscle cell are very important to both training and growth. Remember the muscles use ATP as their fuel for both the growth processes and the muscle contraction process. The body depends on muscle mitochondria to produce its ATP. If not enough ATP is produced in the muscles, the result is muscle fatigue and lower energy levels in the weight room, on the field or on the courts.

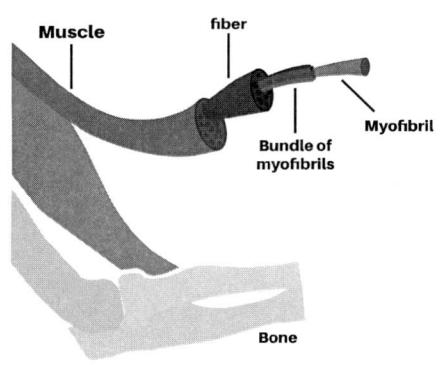

A competitive athlete will spend most of his/her time stimulating the growth, and increasing the number of, myofibrils in the muscle cells. (Myofibrils make up approximately 80 percent of the volume of a muscle fiber.)

Myofibrils are composed of a series of smaller segments called "sarcomeres". A sarcomere literally means "muscle segment." Therefore myofibrils, which are the functional units of skeletal muscle, are made up of a chain of sarcomere units laid end to end, or "in series." This is important to understand and is one of the reasons why it is possible to build up just the lower sections of a muscle group, such as the lower biceps.

Dark and light bands make up each sarcomere and as they spread across a myofibril, they give it the appearance of being striped or striated. The organized stripes are the main elements of each muscle segment, and are responsible for contraction. There are actually two specific types of protein filaments or threads known as "myofiliments".

Myofiliments are composed of "Z-lines" or "Z-Disks", "I" bands, "A" bands, "M" lines, actin and myosin. These are merely descriptive names for the regions of each sarcomere. The two specific protein filaments that make up the sarcomeres and are responsible for contraction is a thin filament called "actin" and the thicker filament is called "myosin".

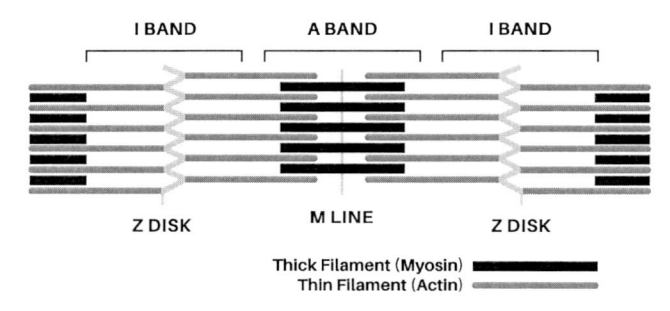

Under the microscope, a muscle myofiliment looks like it is comprised of dark and light colored bands. Early German researchers gave names to these bands and segments. It is the intricate movement of these bands using the energy created by oxygen that causes muscles to contract and relax.

The "A" Band is the darker section of the sarcomeres and this is where the thick myosin filaments extend all the way through the muscle cell and the thin actin filaments extend partway across it. Therefore the "A" Band is where the actin overlaps the myosin proteins. (The "A" actually stands for "Anisotropic", which, in German, means that it "appears darker" as more light is absorbed by these fibers.)

The "I" Band is where only the actin proteins go across the muscle cell and meet each other and where no thick filaments are found. ("I" stands for "Isotropic" in German and means that the area appears to be "lighter" because more light can pass through it.)

The "Z-line" or "Z Disc" is a thin protein sheet that connects the actin filaments to each other and also connects each sarcomere to each other. (The "Z" stands for "Zwishensheibe" which means "between the disk.")

To summarize: the "A" Band is darker because it contains actin and myosin filaments that overlap each other and the "I" Band is lighter in color because the filaments do not overlap each other. This is why a muscle fiber appears striated. Furthermore all the seemingly confusing names for regions of a myofibril/sarcomere are simply labels for those regions based on how the early German scientists saw these regions under a microscope.

How a Muscle Contracts

When magnified, the thick myosin filaments, have tiny heads protruding out of them. These heads, called "myosin heads", make contact with the actin filaments. Think of them as oars coming out of a boat and the actin proteins as the water. When the brain sends the signal for a muscle to contract, the myosin heads pull the actin proteins closer together, which in turn pulls the "Z-Lines" closer together. This shortens or contracts the sarcomeres.

When thousands of these sarcomeres are contracting in a muscle group, the whole muscle shortens and pulls on the bone that it is attached to these muscles in the desired direction. But this cannot happen without ATP energy created by an ample supply of oxygen.

In a relaxed state, the thin filaments of the actin are separated. When the muscle is contracting, the thin actin filaments are sliding toward each other and the thick myosin filaments remain stationary. This causes the distance between the "Z" Lines to decrease. In the most contracted state, the thin filaments overlap one another and the sarcomeres shorten to their smallest size.

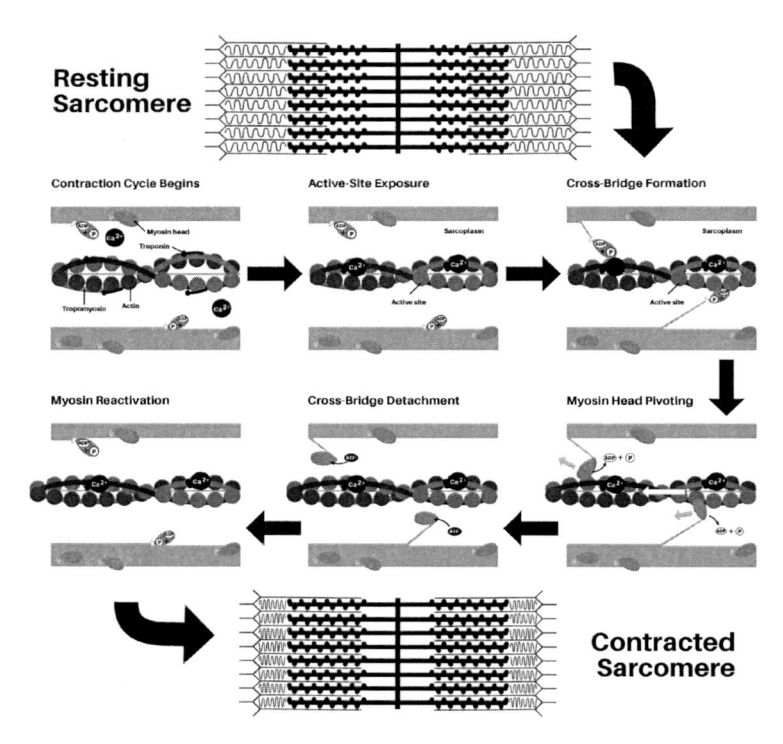

When the brain signals the sarcomere to contract, a rapid set of processes occur in sequence. At each step energy is consumed and waste products are generated before the muscle relaxes once again and awaits it's next signal from the brain.

In order to adapt to repeated and similar contractions, a muscle fiber will multiply the number of myofibrils that it has. More myofibrils improves the muscle's ability to contract and this is accomplished by enlarging the actual size of the fibers. In addition, continued repetitive exercising adds sarcomeres in series to lengthen the myofibrils, The result is bigger and stronger muscles.

Veins, Arteries & Capillaries

As was stated earlier, muscle contraction requires the energy contained within the ATP molecule. In order to synthesize ATP, vital nutrients such as carbohydrates are required, as well as the terminal electron acceptor "oxygen". Metabolic waste products from muscular contraction, as well as other cellular reactions, must also be removed from the muscle cells. This takes oxygen energy.

Muscles require an constant oxygen-rich blood supply to deliver nutrients to the muscle cells. This process is carried out by the blood vessels. Blood vessels are hollow tubes that carry blood. The largest of these are the arteries. They are the largest because they carry blood directly from the heart to the tissues and therefore must withstand high dynamic blood pressures.

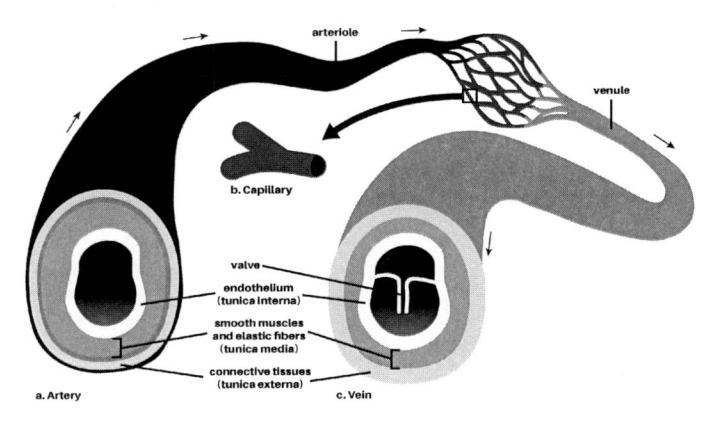

Arteries (a) contain oxygenated blood flowing from the lungs through the heart to the capillaries (b). Veins (c) contain deoxygenated blood heading back to the lungs through the heart.

Capillaries connect each muscle to the cardiovascular system and form channels from the arteries. At some point they become so small that only one red blood cell at a time can pass through the capillary opening and capillaries are so thin that gasses and nutrients can easily permeate the capillary walls.

Veins are the opposite of arteries because they carry deoxygenated blood back to the heart. Hemoglobin, the molecule that carries the oxygen molecules, is red in color when bound to oxygen, When the oxygen is released and the hemoglobin molecules picks up carbon dioxide, the red blood cell takes on a blue color.

Veins are very elastic. They accommodate for blood flow because they actually have muscle cells in the middle of their structure. When blood flow in the veins increases, these muscle cells react to make the veins stronger so they can handle greater blood volume. This is what happens during active physical exertion when more oxygen needs to be delivered to the cells.

Connective Tissue

Muscles contain hundreds and even thousands of fibers. The body arranges them in an organized fashion to form a larger working muscle group (such as the biceps, pecs and quads.) These muscle groups are essential in stabilizing and moving our skeletal system. They are directly, or indirectly, attached to the bone by a specialized group of cells known as "connective tissue" or "fascia".

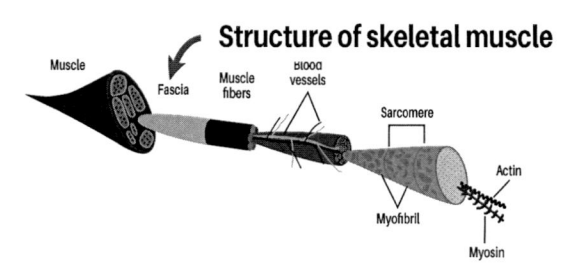

Structure of skeletal muscle

Muscle, Fascia, Muscle fibers, Blood vessels, Sarcomere, Myofibril, Actin, Myosin

The muscle is a complex combination of thousands of fibers, nerves, blood vessels and other tissues each intricately designed to work together to cause a contraction.

Each individual muscle is separated from neighboring muscles and held into place or position by layers of this fascia. In addition to holding a muscle in place, this connective tissue protrudes in a cord-like shape, attaching the muscle group to bone. This extension of the fascia is called a "tendon" or "ligament". Tendons attach, or "bind" our muscles to the bones in the body. Ligaments bind bones together.

How is the skeletal system held together?

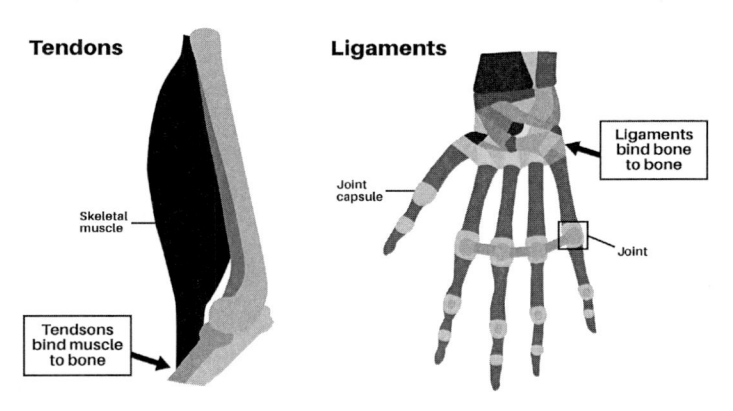

Tendons **Ligaments**

Skeletal muscle

Tendsons bind muscle to bone

Ligaments bind bone to bone

Joint capsule

Joint

Tendons bind our muscles to bones while ligaments bind bones to bones.

The word fascia means "bundle" or "band". Fascia bands tissues and organs together in a collective manner. On a whole, the fascia is a very fibrous, course, flexible, and strong tissue. For example, a tendon, can resist 8,600 to 18,000 pounds per square inch of tension. A muscle's overall ability and function is determined by the arrangement of these fascias. Again, these tissues require a constant supply of oxygen to remain strong.

Oxygen Debt

The additional oxygen that must be taken into an athlete's body after vigorous exercise to help restore all the body's systems back to their normal conditions (or "states") is called the "oxygen debt". Usually, labored breathing can only pay this debt back. This heavy and deep breathing must continue even after exercising has ceased.

Oxygen debt is tied to the build up of the metabolic waste product of muscle contraction known as lactic acid. An accumulation of lactic acid in the muscles creates discomfort, usually muscle cramping, spasms and pain. These symptoms indicate the presence of lactic acid in the muscles. An over-abundance of lactic acid in the muscles can actually interfere with muscle activity. This interference will continue until equilibrium or "homeostasis" is restored and the lactic acid is eliminated from the muscles. This cleansing process takes energy derived from oxygen.

Some of the energy we need to create ATP is generated as the cells break down pyruvic acid. This decomposition process occurs only in the presence of sufficient amounts of oxygen. ATP and oxygen react with pyruvic acid to become carbon dioxide and water.

During exercise, blood vessels in muscles dilate (increase in size) and blood flow is increased in order to supply more oxygen to the muscle cells. Up to a point, the available oxygen is sufficient to meet the energy needs of the body. But, when muscle exertion is high, oxygen cannot be supplied to muscle fibers fast enough, and the aerobic breakdown of pyruvic acid cannot produce enough ATP required for further muscle contraction.

During such periods, additional ATP is generated in a process called "anaerobic[60] glycolysis". In this process, most of the pyruvic acid produced is converted into lactic acid. About 80 percent of this lactic acid diffuses from the

---

[60] Remember "anaerobic" means "in the absence of oxygen".

skeletal muscles into the blood stream and is transported to the liver so it can be converted back into glucose or glycogen. However, some lactic acid continues to accumulate in muscle tissues. More oxygen is required to turn this lactic acid into carbon dioxide and water.

After exercise has stopped, the body needs extra oxygen to continue to metabolize lactic acid wastes, to replenish ATP and to pay back any oxygen debt that has been borrowed from hemoglobin, myoglobin, (an iron-containing substance similar to hemoglobin that is found in muscle fibers,) air in the lungs, and body fluids. Muscle glycogen must also be restored. This is accomplished through diet and may take several days, depending on the intensity of exercise. Athletes call this the "recovery process".

Highly trained athletes can have oxygen requirements that are twice that of average people due to a combination of genetics and training. As a result, they are capable of greater muscle activity without significantly increasing lactic acid production. Their oxygen debts are less. That is why most athletes do not become short of breath as readily as untrained individuals. In any case, the key factor in recovery and overall performance is a consistent supply of oxygen.

Endurance

Endurance plays a major role in every athletic activity. Without endurance training, athletes would not be able to successfully compete in their respective fields. Endurance training involves low resistance and increasing repetitive movements.

Endurance training increases the level of aerobic enzymes which are needed to breakdown carbohydrate fuels to produce energy. Enzymes are proteins that speed up metabolic reactions. They release and transfer energy. Enzymes are influenced by a number of factors. The three most important factors are "temperature", "acidity" and "fuel".

The temperature of the muscles increases as the muscle groups are activated and used. Acidity (lower pH levels) is the result of lactic acid accumulation which in turn reduces enzyme activity and causes muscle fatigue. Enzymes work faster and more efficiently when they have more fuel. The faster the enzyme can breakdown the body's fuel, the faster the muscle can respond and recover.

Endurance training that targets the muscle cells increases the number and size of the mitochondria. As was discussed previously, the mitochondria are the cellular powerhouses that produce energy. All "oxygen" energy production takes place in the mitochondria. So, oxygen is the key to endurance training,

Overall, endurance training appears to fine-tune the body's secretion of, and response to, hormones. This leads to a more efficient use of hormones and energy.

Endurance training affects every part of the body and benefits an athlete physically, mentally and emotionally. Endurance training results in healthier mood state profiles including lower levels of tension, depression, anger, fatigue, and confusion.

Muscle Pain

Theories on the cause of muscle pain and soreness have evolved over the years. In the past, the accumulation of lactic acid was blamed as the primary culprit for aching muscles. However, that theory has changed.

During high levels of physical activity, as the muscles contract, the body does indeed produce lactic acid. This occurs because the muscle's demand for oxygen gets too high and the blood simply cannot deliver all the oxygen the muscles need.

In order to produce energy needed for the muscles to continue to function, the body begins an anaerobic (without oxygen) process to make energy. This anaerobic energy creates even more lactic acid. As this lactic acid builds up and gets trapped inside the muscles, and, because it is an acid, it causes a burning sensation within muscle tissue.

For many years, lactic acid build-up was thought to be the primary cause of sore muscles. Today, we know that this is not totally correct. Research indicates that lactic acid does not remain in the muscles for a long length of time. In fact it takes more than 30 minutes to completely remove lactic acid from muscle tissues after physical exertion.

Since most muscle and joint soreness occurs 24 to 36 hours after exercising, the cause of sore muscles cannot be result of lactic acid being present in the muscles. The real cause for sore muscles is apparently micro-trauma to the muscle fibers. Any physical exertion, whether during work or play, causes some localized damage to the muscle fiber membranes. The damaged muscle becomes inflamed, which causes sore muscles. Damaged muscles also release chemical irritants, which can irritate pain receptors.

The body responds to this damage by increasing blood flow (oxygen) to the localized muscle area. This increased blood flow often causes swelling, which also irritates the pain receptors in the muscles.

Oxygen Relieves Muscle Pain

I have explained how a muscle is constructed, how it functions, and we feel pain pain. The obvious question is "how can we reduce or eliminate the pain caused by tissue inflammation and lactic acid build up?"

If you have read this far into the book, you know the answer is simple: increase the oxygen supply to the muscles and tissues.

The traditional definition of pain is that it is an unpleasant sensation, in varying degrees of severity, as a consequence of injury, disease, or emotional disorder and that causes suffering. There is a growing body of scientific evidence that indicates that the reduction of cellular oxygen can increase pain because the muscles, organs and body systems will no longer function properly.

Dr. C. Samuel West, a specialist in the science of lymphology, and a distinguished member of the international Society of Lymphology, has proven that food present in cells without enough oxygen will turn into waste products (like lactic acid) and fat. He has written that the less oxygen present in the cells, the more pain we experience.[61]

Dr. West is a strong advocate of exercise since a lack of exercise reduces circulation, the transfer of oxygen to the cells and results in high blood pressure and fluid retention. Any one of these conditions will upset the metabolic processes and functioning of the cell. The cells, lacking sufficient oxygen, start manufacturing chemical byproducts and soon the cells, and the surrounding cells, become weak and unhealthy. If prolonged, cellular stress occurs and the organs, as well as the entire immune system, may break down and malfunction allowing conditions where disease organisms can flourish.

The reduction of cellular A.T.P. drastically alters the body's sodium-potassium balance in the individual cells, in the blood stream, and in the fluid that surrounds the cells. The chemical change also alters and reduces the "electrical fields" in the cells, and the blood stream.

Once this electrical change occurs, minerals begin to "fall out" of the fluids surrounding the cells and the bloodstream. These minerals begin sticking or clumping together in what is called "mineral deposits". If these minerals settle in the joints, arthritis occurs; in the eyes, cataracts occur.

---

[61] West, C. Samuel. The Golden Seven Plus One, (Seventh Printing), Utah: Samuel Publishing, April 1988.

When they settle in the arteries, we describe the process as "hardening of the arteries."

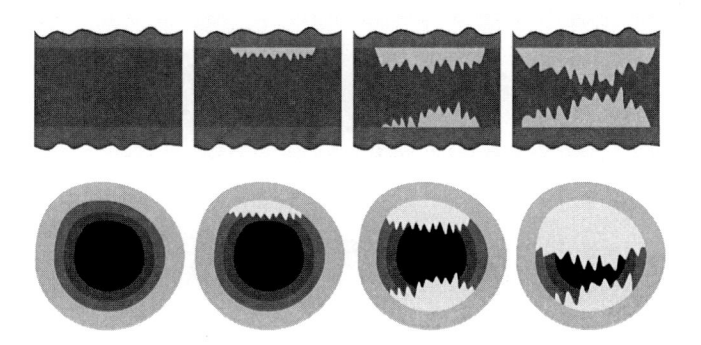

*Top: Cross section of arterial plaque build-up.
Bottom: Cross-section arterial place build-up.*

Our muscles respond to electrical charges sent by the brain. These messages tell the muscles to contract and release. Anything that upsets this delicate and intricate electrical transfer of energy generated by A.T.P., will cause the muscles to spasm or work respond poorly causing discomfort and even extreme levels of pain. Also, prolonged or excessive stress to the muscles, joints or organs in the body causes the body to increase the production of specific hormones designed to relieve the body of pain. (These hormones can include cortisol and epinephrine, which we call adrenaline.) These same hormones, however, cause dramatic changes in metabolism, blood pressure and heart rates.

As the pressure, stress, anxiety or prolonged physical activities increase, these blood hormones become trapped in the tissues. As Dr. Kurt Donsbach, N.D. explains:

> *"These blood proteins attract and retain water in the body tissue, creating a localized edema thus bringing about swelling. The edema will in turn slow down the the distribution of oxygen and the dis-*

posal of carbon dioxide from the cells. The lack of oxygen, the chemicals released from damaged cells, and the pressure to the nerve endings, will create pain. 'Tissue that is inflamed tends to lose flexibility and thus creates an initial stiffness. The stiffness, accumulation of blood proteins, fluids and salts, and the transformation of energy into heat, will precipitate and crystallize substances like calcium and uric acid creating a vicious cycle that culminates with chronic pain and deformities."[62]

---

[62] Donsbach, Kurt, N.D., Ph.D. Embracing Holistic Health. Al-Don Institute of Experimental Medicine, Bonita, CA 1992: 61-62.

Chapter Eight:
Our Diet and Oxygen

> Rubble, garbage, toxins, refuse, debris and anything useless are destroyed by oxygen and carried out of the system. Just as a clean house holds little interest to passing flies, likewise an oxygen rich body is a difficult fortress to assail.
> Brian Goulet, Certified Herbalist
> Canadian Journal of Health and Nutrition

We live in the world of fast-food convenience and instant-gratification. No modern society consumes more red meats and dairy products than does America. Research currently estimates that over 45% of the American diet is fat. Unfortunately, animal and dairy products contain high concentrations of cholesterol. While the body needs some "good" cholesterol to run efficiently, (like those from grains or nuts,) the cholesterol from meats and dairy products passes directly in to the blood stream and begins to "trap" blood proteins which are so important for stabilizing and regulating the flow of oxygen to the cells.

The excessive consumption of cholesterol/fat-ridden food robs oxygen from the blood stream. Fats easily combine with oxygen and form "free radicals". These free radicals use more oxygen to form peroxides that damage and destroy the cells. As far back as 1977, it was reported in the Scientific American (February Issue) that:

> "...cholesterol epoxide (peroxide) and other substances formed from cholesterol will cause cells to mutate and which will cause cancer."[63]

---

[63] McCord, Joe and Findivich, Irwin Superoxides and Superoxide Dismutase. Academic Press, N. Y., 1977. McGaffigan, Patricia A., RN., M.S. "Hazards of Hypoxemia," Nursing, May, 1996.

Fatty foods, which are the major caloric foods consumed by most Americans, cause an oxygen deficiency. This deficiency causes a cascade in deteriorating physiological conditions that increase our disease potential . Cancer is only one such a disease.

We know that cells that lose their ability to utilize oxygen can become cancerous.[64] These cells have been oxygen-starved for so long that they undergo a metabolic "shift" and revert to a metabolism that does not use oxygen as the spark for cellular respiration (called anaerobic metabolism).

This is, of course, the ultimate and last state of cellular degeneration which is caused by a low oxygen life-style. It is also interesting that research shows that people who consume very high quantities of fat have a far greater incidence of cancer as well as other degenerative diseases. Thus, cholesterol rich foods, (those lacking the life-giving oxygen found in raw vegetables, etc., which are easily converted into energy,) are converted into toxic waste and fat in the cells.

The toxic waste and fat in the cells impedes the nutrient supply to the cells from the blood stream. In addition, all the current nutritional research clearly indicates that foods high in sugars, salts, fats and cholesterol are directly responsible for problems like kidney and heart diseases, liver damage, high blood pressure, hardening of the arteries, obesity, and strokes. Dr. Levine has described the consequences of cellular oxygen deficiencies in this way: it is

> "...an acidic condition, caused by the the accumulation of acidic by-products, occurs in poorly oxygenated cells. Soft drinks, caffeine, alcohol, and red meats are among the substances that cause

---

[64] See Dr. Warburg's lecture notes in Appendix Four for more detailed information on the relationship of cancer and low oxygen levels,

> systemic (whole body) acidity where there is an excess of positively charged hydrogen ions (H$^+$)."[65]

When excessive amounts of hydrogen ions are in the tissues they will combine with, (and thus utilize,) oxygen resulting in an oxygen deficient state.

> "When cells are deprived of oxygen, lactic acid accumulates and the cellular environment becomes acidic. This reduces available oxygen for the primary function of metabolism because more oxygen is needed to neutralize the acid."[66]

Meat and dairy foods, which are high in cholesterol, break down (digest) in our stomach and intestines. These foods are potentially harmful if consumed in excess since their chemical by-products dilate (widen or expand) the capillaries making the distance that the water has to travel to and from the cells much greater.

The greater the distance that the fluids must travel, in the same amount of time, the less the transfer of nutrients, oxygen and minerals to the cells. Also the less toxins, waste products, poisons, etc. are transferred back out of the cells and in to the blood stream. These waste products begin to accumulate in the cells. Stretched capillary walls allow the blood proteins to escape and lodge themselves between the cells.

The trapped proteins permit the accumulation of excess fluids around the cells. This prevents the cells from getting the very oxygen they need and so the glucose begins to ferment resulting in electrical changes within the cells.

Oxygen rich red blood cells carry a negative electrical charge. They travel through the capillaries single file. As the capillaries dilate, and the electrical balance of our body

---

[65] op. cit. Levine and Kidd, "Antioxidant Adaptation"

[66] ibid.

changes because of a lack of oxygen, these blood cells are now dispersed over a greater volume in the capillaries and it becomes more difficult for them to travel the now greater distances to the cells,

To further complicate matters, the red blood cells, because of the electrical change, begin to clump together and cause a microscopic traffic jam in the capillaries. This further dilates the capillaries and allows more blood proteins to escape and lodge in the spaces around the cells. This produces more fluid around the cells and the process repeats itself until the cells begin to die because of lack of oxygen.

Individuals eating diets high in fat intake seriously affect the immune system's ability to compensate for the increased amounts of toxins in the blood stream. Increased levels of toxins create conditions where pathogenic microorganisms can thrive. These micro-organisms release additional toxic wastes that the body is now forced to metabolize and eliminate to prevent additional poisoning of the cells.

Because fats and toxins rob oxygen from the body, the body's oxygen levels continue to decline. As the levels decline, cellular respiration (energy production), which requires oxygen, becomes less efficient and more waste products and toxins accumulate both inside and outside the cells. Soon, as the body attempts to adapt to these low oxygen levels to survive, the entire body is so deprived of oxygen that only the most vital organ functions get the available oxygen, with the brain and heart muscles receiving the lion's share,

This extreme oxygen-deprived condition is called "hypoxemia" and the result of prolonged low tissue oxygenation is tissue damage and even cell death. Patricia A. Mc-

Gaffigan, R.N., M.S., identified five major causes of hypoxemia in her article "Hazards of Hypoxemia".[67]

> "Contrary to many medical professionals beliefs, only low levels of "inspired" oxygen are available to individuals at very high altitudes. While the body does adapt itself to this change in atmospheric pressure, the fact is that less oxygen is consumed reducing the effectiveness of the body's respiratory and metabolic functioning. Prolonged high-altitude conditions, like those experienced by mountain climbers, can result in temporary brain damage and even death.
>
> "Conditions which prevent full lung ventilation can affect the body's ability to reach optimum blood oxygen saturation. These conditions can include neurological diseases, the effect of narcotics on the nervous and musculature system, musculoskeletal disorders that prevent the proper functioning of the respiratory muscles, respiratory obstructions or scar tissue damage to the lungs as a result of diseases like chronic bronchitis, pneumonia, asthma, smoking or other toxic fumes or gasses which damage the alveoli in the lungs.
>
> "The membranes which permit the passing of oxygen and carbon dioxide between the capillaries and the alveoli may become thicker. This can be caused by diseases like chronic bronchitis, pneumonia, asthma, fibrosis, pulmonary edema, smoking or other toxic fumes or gasses.
>
> "Poor pulmonary circulation can and does reduce oxygen distribution in the body. This occurs because of a variety of disorders including damaged capillaries and arterial plaque build-up.
>
> "Lower blood oxygen levels can be the result of anemia disorders, sleep apnea, those suffering from

---

[67] McCord, Joe and Findivich, Irwin Superoxides and Superoxide Dismutase. Academic Press, N. Y., 1977. McGaffigan, Patricia A., RN., M.S. "Hazards of Hypoxemia," Nursing, May, 1996.

upper abdominal or thoracic pain resulting in shallow breathing and carbon monoxide poisoning."

While Ms. McGaffigan points out that some of the causes of hypoxemia are medical or genetic abnormalities, many of the causes are dietary related. Poor nutrition is at the heart of most degenerative problems that prevent the uptake and utilization of life-giving oxygen. Certainly an improved diet and regular exercise will enhance overall health and oxygenation and must not be overlooked nor minimized. However, supplemental oxygen (oxygen therapies) can also help in bringing the body back to its normal, healthy state. As Ms. McGaffigan confirms:

> *"You can administer supplemental oxygen by various methods and at different doses depending on the patient's degree of hypoxemia."*[68]

Dr. Stephen Levine, Ph.D. summarized the conditions leading to a condition of hypoxemia in this manner:

> *"In all serious disease states, we find a concomitant low oxygen state. Low oxygen in the body is a sure indicator for disease. Hypoxemia, or lack of oxygen in the tissues, is the fundamental cause of all degenerative disease."* [69]

---

[68] Ibid.

[69] op.cit. Levine and Kidd, "Antioxidant Adaptation"

Chapter Nine:
The Skin:
Oxygen for the
Body's Largest Organ

Skin is the great protector. Its outer layer, the epidermis, is thinner than Saran Wrap; it is stain-resistant and waterproof. Tightly woven epidermal cells form a sturdy barrier to hold moisture in as well as keep unwanted water out. On the surface, dead, compacted, and sloughing cells add toughness, a kind of see-through coat of armor. With a cleverness the military would envy, the epidermis brims with stem cells ready to spin out reinforcements as needed, and pigment-producing melanocytes deflect skin's No. 1 enemy--the sun. Its rays are especially damning to the skin's middle layer, the dermis. Indeed, the skin is a powerful interface between the mind, the body, and the external world...The skin also has a rich life as an endocrine organ, manufacturing hormones like vitamin D for the rest of the body, and steroids and thyroid hormone for its own use. Though it's not always clear why, the skin makes many of the neurotransmitters and hormones found in the brain.[70]

The skin is a natural wonder whose complexity is partially indicated by the fact that our skin covers an average of nineteen square feet yet weighs less than seven pounds. A cross section reveals three well-defined layers.

The epidermis is the outermost layer known as the cuticle or protective layer. It is made of tightly packed, scale-like cells that are continually being shed. An entirely new epidermal cuticle layer of skin forms every twenty-eight days. (Though this is cycle slows down as we age.)

---

[70] "Skin Deep; As the body's largest organ, skin is a powerful yet unappreciated veneer'", Bernadine Healy, M.D., June 24, 2013 U.S. News and World Report.
http://health.usnews.com/usnews/health/articles/051114/14skin.htm

The next layer is the dermis. It is also called the 'true skin' because most of the vital functions of the skin are performed in this layer. The dermis contains the glands that secrete perspiration and sebum (oil), the papilla (hair manufacturing plants), nerve fibers, blood vessels, lymph glands and sense receptors. The dermis has an elastic quality because it contains the protein connective tissues called elastin and collagen[71]. These proteins give skin its strength as well as its flexibility.

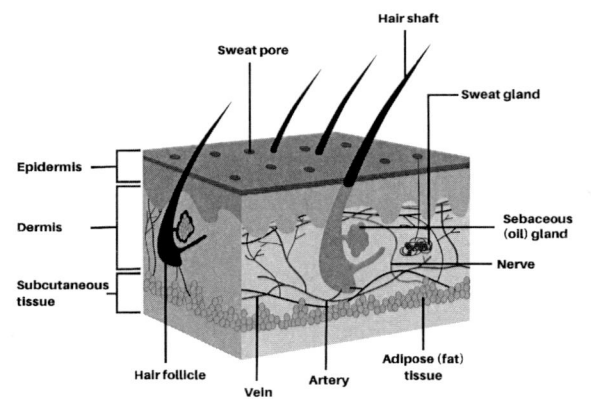

A cross section of human skin.

Below the dermis is the third layer called the subcutaneous layer. It is made of a fatty tissue that gives skin its smoothness, contour and serves as a shock absorber for

---

[71] Collagen is the protein that holds the body together. It is the most abundant protein of the body, making up 25%–35% of the body's protein content. It is a key component in blood vessels, the corneas in the eyes, cartilage, skin, muscles, tendons, bones and the connective tissues. It provides strength and structure and it plays an important part in the healing, repair and skin regeneration process, and is responsible for the production of new skin cells. Elastin is another protein found in the connective tissues. It helps the body resume its form after contracting or expanding. Elastin helps the tissues remain elastic. Apart from giving the skin a healthy and young look, elastin is also the protein that lines blood vessels and arteries, allowing them to adjust to variations of blood pressure throughout the day. Elastin also permits the lungs to expand as well as the bladder and elastic cartilage.

the vital organs. In addition, this layer stores the energy made by oxygen metabolism and acts an effective body insulator.

Together, these three layers form the 'living fabric' known as skin. In one square inch of skin there are about 65 hairs, 100 sebaceous (oil) glands, 234 feet of nerves, 60 feet of blood vessels, 650 sweat glands, 1,300 nerve endings, twenty sebaceous glands, 19,500 sensory cells at the ends of nerve fibers, 80 cold detection nerve endings and 165 pressure sensors.

Unbroken, the skin is our first line of defense against disease and bacterial invasion. It regulates body temperatures, sends neurological messages to the brain, detoxifies the body by excreting wastes (as sweat), respires (absorbs oxygen and releases carbon dioxide), absorbs nutrients, manufactures Vitamin D and protects the body from ultra violet (UV) damage from the sun.

The skin actually takes in oxygen and expels carbon dioxide. In fact, the skin does up to 5 percent or more of all the "breathing" done by the body[72]. The skin, as an important organ, also functions just like the kidneys because the skin eliminates about two pints of water and salts every single day.

Our skin needs a consistent supply of oxygen to stay young and healthy, just like every other cell in our bodies. The skin needs oxygen to survive, reproduce, and regenerate healthy tissue. We know that the most common cause of aging is an oxygen deficiency at the cellular level. So, when our skin does not get a sufficient amount of oxygen,

---

[72] "It has been known since 1851 that atmospheric oxygen is taken up by the human epidermis. The contribution to total respiration is negligible...In this study it has been shown that under normal conditions, atmospheric oxygen can supply the upper skin layers to a depth of 0.25–0.40 mm. This is 3–10 times deeper than has been calculated previously. The whole epidermis and the upper corium can therefore be supplied with oxygen from the atmosphere." Fitzgerald, 1957; Baumgärtl et al. 1987.

it prematurely ages, loses firmness, elasticity and becomes pale in color.

The skin renews itself every four weeks and is very responsive to what goes on the inside of the body. Makeup can cover some signs of an unhealthy life-style, but ultimately a poor diet, smoking, excessive alcohol consumption, use of recreational drugs, and the resulting free radical damage will become apparent no matter how good the makeup job is. The quality and health of our skin reflects the quality of the raw materials used to make up its cells.

Most skin-care products on the market today are "cosmetic cover-ups," which means they cover-up skin problems. Many skin care products contain ingredients that suffocate the skin by keeping oxygen out and trap in toxins. Just remember that the skin needs oxygen to breathe, and oxygen keeps the skin strong, healthy, and looking young.

Throughout the course of our lives, our skin will change. It will change from the soft and delicate characteristics of baby skin to childhood's smooth, velvety texture and resilience. During the teenage years, the skin reacts to changes in our diets and hormones and continues to change through the twenties when our skin begins to finally mature. By our thirties, the skin begins drying and we notice signs of the first wrinkles. By forty, our skin is aging. As the skin ages, it characteristically becomes drier and loses its elasticity.

As we age, the skin's rejuvenating capacity slows down and the oxygen and nutrient supply to the skin decreases due to a decrease in blood circulation. Protective oil (sebum) production declines. These changes take place in the dermal layer of the skin. Just how fast, and to what extent, this dermal layer changes depends on three things: our age, our heredity (genetics) and lifestyle.

Ongoing research has determined that, as we get older, the ability of our skin to absorb and utilize oxygen declines. Our skin tissue loses about 30% of its oxygen "capacity" by the age of 30 and close to 60% by age 40. As oxygen metabolism decreases, the cells cannot dispose of wastes and cannot fully utilize key molecules in the blood stream. Therefore, free-radical damage increases dramatically as we get older.

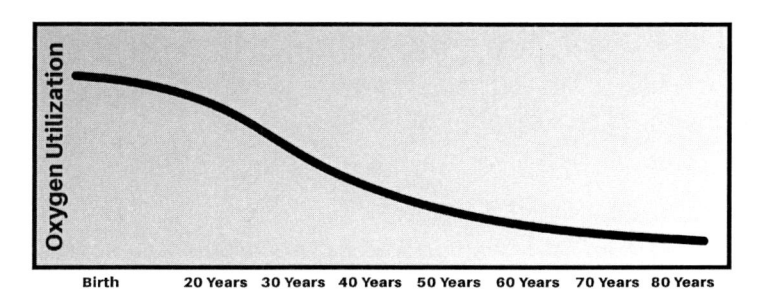

Skin requires oxygen to look and feel healthy. As we grow older, the skin's ability to use oxygen declines.

On the surface of aging skin, the cells work their way from the dermal layer outward These cells become thicker and more dense and lose their ability to retain moisture. Lubrication (oil) decreases, which gives mature skin its dry, scaly appearance.

Remember that the body consists of more than 70 percent water and some skin cells contain over 90 percent water. When cells lose water, they diminish in size and flatten out. Then they lose their capacity to absorb oxygen for vital metabolic functions. Chronic cell dehydration appears as lines, wrinkles and lackluster skin.

Parched and dehydrated skin is unable to retain moisture. It usually feels "tight" and uncomfortable after washing, unless some type of moisturizer or skin cream is applied. Chapping and cracking are signs of extremely dry and dehydrated skin.

Dryness is further exacerbated by wind, temperature and air-conditioning, all of which cause the skin to flake, chap and feel tight. Tight skin is drawn over bones. It looks dull, especially on the cheeks and around the eyes. Tiny "expression lines" appear at the corners of the mouth and eyes.

The topical application of oxygen-enhanced skin-care products may dramatically improve skin health by promoting blood flow and enhancing moisture retention. Exfoliating, or sloughing off dead cells, also boosts circulation to the surface of the skin, imparting a rosy glow. Removing dead cells on the surface of the skin also improves the skin's ability to absorb oxygen and nutrients.

Chapter Ten:
Drugs, Disease & the Immune System

The link between insufficient oxygen and disease has now been firmly established.
Dr. W. Spencer Way, M.D.
The Journal of the American Association of Physicians

Most individuals when they become "sick" turn to conventional medicines to correct the problem. These approaches include prescription drugs, over-the-counter drugs, radiation, chemical (chemo) therapies, and surgery. Researchers have learned, however, that many traditional approaches to address illness have serious side-effects, not the least of which is accidental death.

Prescription medications deplete the body of oxygen as energy is required to convert these chemicals into compounds that the body can either use or dispose of in some manner. In fact, before we take a look at the real effect drugs have had on our immune system, consider these alarming statistics:

- In 2015, 4.06 billion prescriptions were written by doctors. That is an average of 13 prescriptions for every man, woman and child in America. That is more than one drug prescription every month.[73]
- In 2007, the Journal of the American Medical Association (JAMA) wrote that prescription drugs were the

---

[73] Prescription drug abuse is a global problem, and the U.S. is the world's biggest addict. Americans account for 99 percent of the world's hydrocodone (Vicodin) consumption, 80 percent of the world's oxycodone (Percocet and Oxycontin) consumption and 65 percent of the world's hydromorphone (Dilaudid) consumption, according to the New York Times.
https://www.drugwatch.com/2015/07/29/drug-abuse-in-america/

second leading cause of accidental death in the U.S.. By 2011, it had replaced auto deaths and became number one.[74]

- In 2014, 47,055 people died from drug overdoses -- 1.5 times greater than the number killed in car crashes.
- Opioids are involved in 61% of all drug overdose deaths. The latest CDC data finds that deaths from natural opiates such as morphine, codeine and semi-synthetic prescription pain killers like oxycodone and hydrocodone jumped 10% from 2013 to 2014.
- Deaths from heroin overdoses rose 26%. The biggest increase in deaths was from from synthetic opioids, which went up 80%. According to the CDC, the increase in synthetic opioid deaths coincided with increased reports by law enforcement of illicitly manufactured fentanyl.[75]
- In the United Kingdom, it is estimated that the number of prescription pills that each citizen takes during his/her lifetime amounts to more than 14,000 pills. "...Including over-the-counter drugs, the 14,000 number would swell to 40,000 pills taken in a lifetime. What are the effects of all these drugs? We are looking at a supreme Trojan Horse that is rotting out America and other industrialized countries from the inside. Wars, no wars, economic deprivation, economic prosperity, the drugs continue to do their work, debilitating and ruining and terminating lives."[76]

---

[74] Unintentional Poisoning Deaths—United States, 1999-2004 JAMA. 2007;297(12):1309-1311. doi:10.1001/jama.297.12.1309.

[75] http://www.cnn.com/2015/12/18/health/drug-overdose-deaths-2014

[76] http://jonrappoport.wordpress.com/2012/09/15/shocker-how-many-drug-prescriptions-are-written-in-the-us-every-year/trackback/

In another CDC finding, it was observed that:

> *"Experts say that doctors are sometimes quick to prescribe antibiotics for all sorts of symptoms, even though antibiotics work only against bacterial infections, not against viruses such as the flu or the common cold. More than 50 million of the 150 million antibiotic prescriptions written each year for patients outside of hospitals are unnecessary."*[77]

The Rise of the Super Bugs:

Antibiotics have indeed been effective in removing many pathogenic bacteria from our bodies. Many lives have been saved by using penicillin as well as other antibiotics in combating bacterial infections.

However, traditional antibiotic approaches are no longer as effective as they once were. Many bacteria have become resistant to our arsenal of drug ammunition. As fast as pharmaceutical companies come up with new drugs to fight new strains of these organisms, the strains mutate, change their cellular and metabolic structures, become stronger, more resilient and present a new dreadful challenge to the medical community. In fact, bacteria even transfer genes among themselves increasing their resistance to specialized drugs.

Currently, there are over 100 different antibiotics in existence. Unfortunately, there is always at least one strain of microorganism that resists one or more of these wonder drugs. Why?

More and more research is pointing to the proliferation and easy access to prescription drugs (antibiotics) and the repeated and the extensive use of these antibiotics as the single most significant factor in the mutation of micro-organisms. Many even blame the drug industry itself. With its

---

[77] Conly J, Johnston B. Where are all the new antibiotics? The new antibiotic paradox. Can J Infect Dis Med Microbiol. 2005 May;16(3):159-60.

desire for more profits, access to prescription and over-the-counter formulations is easier to obtain than at any time in our nation's history. Consumers pop pills like they are candy. Whenever we get an ache, pain, feel uncomfortable, etc., we take another pill. But for every cause there is an inevitable reaction. For bacteria, this reaction is called "resistance".

The more pills and antibiotics we consume, the weaker our immune system gets. As bacteria are assaulted by these drugs, a few survive the battle because the drugs are selective. If only a few bacteria remain resistant, they immediately regroup and become a greater menace to the body.

The World Health Organization (W.H.O.) reported that over 4.3 million people die of respiratory infections every year, primarily from pneumonia. The New England Journal of Medicine reported a new outbreak of whooping cough in 1993. In 1994, Time Magazine reported a resistant cholera epidemic that killed over 50,000 people in Rwanda.[78]

There are other infectious diseases that are resisting current prescription drugs. Lyme disease has stricken more than 150,000 Americans since it was discovered in 1976 and each year the CDC reports another 30,000 new cases. A Bengal cholera strain killed over 5,000 people in Bangladesh not to mention tens of thousands that became seriously ill. E. coli O157 is a food bacteria that killed two and sickened over 500 people who ate at Jack-in-the-Box Restaurants in the U.S. during the late 1990s. In Japan, the same bacteria sickened over 10,000 people. This bacteria has now become one of the leading causes of kidney failure in children today.[79] ABC News reported:

---

[78] The actual reported death toll was 65,66,67.

[79] -- "Exotic diseases are sounding alarms", Telegram Tribune, Jan. 3, 1995; 1. "Staph germ becoming unstoppable", Telegram Tribune, Tues. May 29, 1997: 1.

"The swine flu virus, H1N1, may have killed 15 times the number of people counted by the World Health Organization, according to a new study. And unlike the seasonal flu, the H1N1 pandemic struck down mostly young people, many living in Africa and Southeast Asia. Beginning in 2009, the virus swept the globe, and the WHO counted 18,500 swine flu deaths that had been confirmed by laboratory tests. But according to new estimates from researchers at the U.S. Centers for Disease Control and Prevention, the virus probably killed between 105,700 and 400,000 people around the world in its first year alone, and an additional 46,000 to 179,000 people likely died of cardiovascular complications from the virus."[80]

Here is one common example quoted from a recent Associated Press news release that explains the challenges facing medical practitioners today:

"A staph germ that causes thousands of often deadly infections among hospital patients each year is becoming resistant to medicine's drug of last resort and could soon prove unstoppable. A new strain of Staphylococcus areus bacteria that was discovered in a Japanese infant showed resistance for the first time against vancomycin, which has been around since 1970 and is used when other antibiotics fail...Doctors have long known that many common bacteria are growing resistant to antibiotics. The resistance is attributed to the overuse of antibiotics and the failure of some patients to take their medicine properly. "Penicillin was a wonder drug that killed staph germs when it became available in 1947. Within a decade, some strains grew

---

[80] H1N1 Swine Flu May Have Killed 15 Times More Than First Said. Carrie Gann. ABC News Medical Unit, June 25, 2012, http://abcnews.go.com/Health/swine-flu-h1n1-pandemic-deaths-15-times-higher/story?id=16646281

resistant. Then came methicillin in the 1960s, then vancomycin, which was so potent it was regarded as medicine's 'silver bullet' against staph. "'We have been living since 1970 using vancomycin with no fear that any staph was going to be resistant to it' said Dr. Robert Haley, chief of epidemiology at University of Texas Southwestern Medical Center in Dallas and former chief of C.D.C.'s (Center for Disease Control) hospital infections branch. This changes the whole game."[81]

Each week more examples are appearing in dozens of major publications indicating clearly that both the medical profession and the pharmaceutical companies are losing the battle against disease organisms. This again is contrary to the belief that we are eradicating disease from modern society. We need to heed the warnings from the CDC that the overuse of prescription drugs can harm us in ways that we simply cannot comprehend.

"Antibiotics and similar drugs, together called antimicrobial agents, have been used for the last 70 years to treat patients who have infectious diseases. Since the 1940s, these drugs have greatly reduced illness and death from infectious diseases. However, these drugs have been used so widely and for so long that the infectious organisms the antibiotics are designed to kill have adapted to them, making the drugs less effective. Each year in the United States, at least 2 million people become infected with bacteria that are resistant to antibiotics and at least 23,000 people die each year as a direct result of these infections."[82]

---

[81] -- "Exotic diseases are sounding alarms", Washington (AP), Telegram Tribune, Jan. 3, 1995; 1.

[82] https://www.cdc.gov/drugresistance/

By the way, humans are not the only ones taking antibiotics. Cows, chickens, pigs, cattle, sheep, ducks and other livestock receive doses on a regular basis to reduce mortality and to shorten the time it takes to get meat to market. This widespread and non-discriminate use of antibiotics and hormones adds to the global selective pressure upon bacterial populations.

> *"Approximately 80 percent of the antibiotics sold in the United States are used in meat and poultry production...A key question is, can antibiotic use in animals promote the development of hard-to-treat antibiotic-resistant superbugs that make people sick? And if it can, are the illnesses rare occurrences, and the risks theoretical, or could current usage in animals pose a serious threat to human health...But Consumers Union has concluded that the threat to public health from the overuse of antibiotics in food animals is real and growing. Humans are at risk both due to potential presence of superbugs in meat and poultry, and to the general migration of superbugs into the environment, where they can transmit their genetic immunity to antibiotics to other bacteria, including bacteria that make people sick. Numerous health organizations, including the American Medical Association, American Public Health Association, Infectious Disease Society of America, and the World Health Organization, agree and have called for significant reductions in the use of antibiotics for animal food production. Scientific expert bodies for more than two decades have concluded that there is a connection between antibiotic use in animals and the loss of effectiveness of these drugs in human medicine."*[83]

---

[83] The Overuse of Antibiotics in Food Animals Threatens Public Health http://consumersunion.org/news/the-overuse-of-antibiotics-in-food-animals-threatens-public-health-2/

Salmonella infections are becoming more deadly primarily due to the antibiotic treatment of animals. Unregulated livestock antibiotic usage is altering the animals' bacterial flora. When we consume the meat and by-products from these animals (cheese, milk, eggs, etc.), we increase the concentration, and the effect, of these chemicals in our own bodies. This causes stress to our organs and depletes our bodies of oxygen.

As Streptococcus A receded in its proliferation, Streptococcus B stepped into its place in bacterial ecology. Strep A mutated and multiplied behind the scenes until it made headlines in the 1980s. Then it began striking people of all ages and all classes, almost at random. In 1989 it claimed its most famous victim, Jim Henson, the creator of the Muppets. Many remember toxic shock syndrome (TSS) which was associated with Tampons. This infection was a resistant strain of the Strep A, bacterium.[84]

We know that when we kill germs with antibiotics, a few germs survive. The germs that survive are tougher than the germs that were killed. When we use antibiotics all the time, we create evolutionary pressure. The surviving germs reproduce and pass their genes for "toughness" (or resistance) on to the next generation.

Germs measure their generations in minutes. Strep and staph, two of the most common bacteria, can produce multiple generations with a matter of hours. That means 20,000 or 50,000 generations of strep are produced for

---

[84] TSS is a complication arising from infection from certain types of bacteria and an adverse bodily response to the toxins they produce. TSS from S. aureus has a mortality rate of between 5 and 15 percent, but for streptococcal TSS, the mortality rate jumps up to 30 to 70 percent.
"Women are still getting Toxic Shock Syndrome, and no one quite knows why"
https://www.washingtonpost.com/news/speaking-of-science/wp/2016/03/21/women-are-still-getting-toxic-shock-syndrome-and-no-one-quite-knows-why/?utm_term=.d51897cab740

every one human generation. Bacteria also mutate much more easily than humans.

Stated another way: a standard laboratory bacterium divides into two new cells in the course of twenty to thirty minutes, and these two cells are each immediately ready to grow and divide into two more cells in the next twenty minutes. A single bacterium therefore can produce almost 70 billion cells in the course of twelve hours. A single cell, left unrestrained, can reproduce itself in sheer volume in just 24 hours to fill 15 Olympic swimming pools with each pool containing 660,000 gallons of bacteria.

Time	Increase in the number of cells
0 Minutes	1 (2^0)
20 Minutes	2 (2^1)
40 Minutes	4 (2^2)
60 Minutes	8 (2^3)
80 Minutes	16 (2^4)
100 Minutes	32 (2^5)
120 Minutes	64 (2^6)
3 Hours	512 (2^9)
4 Hours	4,096 (2^{12})
8 Hours	16,777,216 (2^{24})
12 Hours	68,719,476,736 (2^{36})

Some bacteria reproduce so quickly that they can replicate themselves from one single cell to almost 70 billion cells in less than 12 hours.

Some bacteria have another technique for dealing with threats to their existence: sporulation. When exposed to a toxic environment, they go dormant, toughening their cell walls to a nearly impermeable state, to wait until conditions improve. Historically, spore formation was a defense against dehydration, high temperatures or other change in the environment. As spores, microbes can drift about unharmed in 'antiseptic' solutions specifically designed to kill them. That is why even 'cold sterilization' is no longer acceptable in dental offices. Dry heat or autoclaving is now virtually mandatory.

In an article in "People" magazine titled "Bad Bad Bugs"[85], the writer reflects the growing concern of Dr. Mitchell Cohen, Director of the Division of Bacterial and Mycotic Diseases of the National Center for Infectious Disease of the Centers for Disease Control and Prevention in Atlanta, Georgia. The article states:

> *"In time, improper handling of antibiotics and natural evolution conspired to allow bacteria to adapt in order to defend themselves against antibiotics. 'Bacteria have a tremendous evolutionary advantage; says Cohen. They reproduce a lot quicker than we do, and there are a lot more of them.' As a result, bacterial diseases thought to be virtually dormant, such as tuberculosis, meningitis and salmonella, have reappeared in recent years in new drug-resistant forms. Viral diseases, such as various flu strains, HIV and the newly discovered and potentially deadly hepatitis C, are resistant to antibiotics and also pose new challenges to researchers."*[86]

The overuse and misuse of antibiotics brings back memories of the earlier part of the 1900s when contracting an infectious disease was like receiving a death sentence. "It's not that too many antibiotics have led us astray," wrote Dr. Jeffrey Fisher, M.D., author of The Plague Makers. "It's the inappropriate use of antibiotics" that has brought on

---

[85] November 9, 1998

[86] Sider.Don. "Every Day, Warns Dr. Mitchell Cohen, More and More Bacteria Are Learning to Look at Antibiotics and Laugh". November 09, 1998, Vol. 50, No. 17

the dangerous propagation of resistant strains of bacteria. This is not a new phenomenon. It has existed since the early 1940s when penicillin first came on the market.[87]

A number of studies indicate that the recent drastic increase in Candida albicans yeast infections is primarily due to the widespread use of antibiotics and the resulting decline in available body oxygen. Candida, a pathogenic yeast that proliferates in the urinary tracts of women, has become resistant to most antibiotics and now infects many of the body's other internal organs (systemic infection) of both men and women. Dr. Stephen Levine wrote:

> *Hypoxia in the patient is a major contributing factor to yeast susceptibility...Adequate cellular oxygenation is therefore critical to cell-mediated immunity...However, the single most important substance for life -- oxygen -- may be the most powerful immune stimulant of all.* [88]

Another concern of medical professionals is that many antibiotics may also remove beneficial as well as pathogenic bacteria. This situation creates an imbalance which promotes an overgrowth of Candida as well as other detrimental organisms. Therefore, when we use antibiotics, we make a tradeoff. We often sacrifice our beneficial bacteria to rid ourselves of the pathogenic bacteria.

When the body encounters pathogens, (like viruses, fungi, bacteria, etc.,) in the blood stream, or in tissues, the immune system's white blood cells surround or "engulf" these invaders. They then bombard these pathogens with self-generated free-radicals, called "superoxides." These

---

[87] -- "Exotic diseases are sounding alarms", Washington (AP), Telegram Tribune, Jan. 3, 1995; 1.

[88] Levine, Dr. Stephen and Kidd, Dr. Parris M. (co-authors): "Antioxidant Adaptation" and "Immunity, Cancer, Oxygen, and Candida Albicans". Let's Live, August, 1986.

"superoxides" are manufactured in the white blood cells using the oxygen they get from the blood stream.

If the immune system is working properly, it will generate more anti-oxidant enzymes to remove the free-radicals to protect the surrounding tissues. The importance of this anti-oxidant defense system cannot be overstated. Without it, the immune system actually works against the body by generating too many free radicals which could damage surrounding tissues and our bodies. If the immune system is stressed, because it is constantly dealing with drug-resistant microorganisms, the system will falter, The body will not be able to keep up with this unrestricted and uncontrolled growth and proliferation of these drug-resistant strains.

Although there are other factors, this breakdown in the immune system is a key factor in allowing the spread of auto-immune diseases like lupus and rheumatoid arthritis. Dr. Hans Kugler, Ph.D., a well-respected research scientist that has monitored the critical link between toxins and compromised immune system functions, reported in Preventative Medicine Update[89] that over the last 40 years our immune systems have declined in their effectiveness against disease by more than 50%. He also points out that toxic chemicals damage our reproductive organs, especially pesticides used on fruits and vegetables. These chemicals are "hormone disrupters" that mimic female estrogen and block the production of testosterone. Dr. Kugler describes this as:

> "...the interaction between a handicapped immune system and the rise in many cancers, the sudden appearance of new and previously unknown diseases - and most likely -- other diseases that are immune related."[90]

---

[89] Kugler, Dr. Hans, Ph.D. Preventative Medicine Update, March, 1988.

[90] ibid.

Now, this book is not about the pros and cons of using prescription or over-the-counter drugs. But it is about how indiscriminately taking these chemicals affects our immune system and depletes our bodies of oxygen.

In addition to the increased immunity to antibiotics by so many diseases that were controllable in the past, a host of new microbial infections are being transmitted between species. Historically, the spread of inter-species related diseases was very small and relatively rare. But the rise of drug-resistant microorganisms is exacerbated by microorganisms that once only infected non-humans.

This inter-species transmission is called "zoonosis". It occurs when an infectious disease is transmitted between species from animals to humans or from humans to animals. In direct zoonosis the disease agent needs only one host for completion of its life cycle without a significant change in the organism during the infected transmission.[91]

In a systematic review of 1,415 pathogens known to infect humans, 61% were zoonotic.[92] This emergence of a pathogen into a new host species is called "disease invasion" or "disease emergence".

HIV is believed to have originated in the monkey kingdom and has killed and infected tens of millions of individuals all over the world. The West Nile virus, spread by mosquitos, appeared in the United States in 1999 in the New York City area, and moved through the country in the summer of 2002 and continues to cause a great amount of illness. Bubonic plague is a zoonotic disease (spread by fleas). Salmonella is spread by contaminated food

---

[91] Maria Cheng, AP Medical Writer.
<http://hosted.ap.org/dynamic/stories/E/EU_MED_TWO_DISEASES_QA?SITE=AP&SECTION=HOME&TEMPLATE=DEFAULT&CTIME=2013-05-13-09-34-16>

[92] Taylor et al. 2001 Risk factors for human disease emergence Philosophical Transactions of the Royal Society B 356(1411):983-9

supplies.[93] Rocky Mountain spotted fever and Lyme disease[94] are spread by infected ticks.

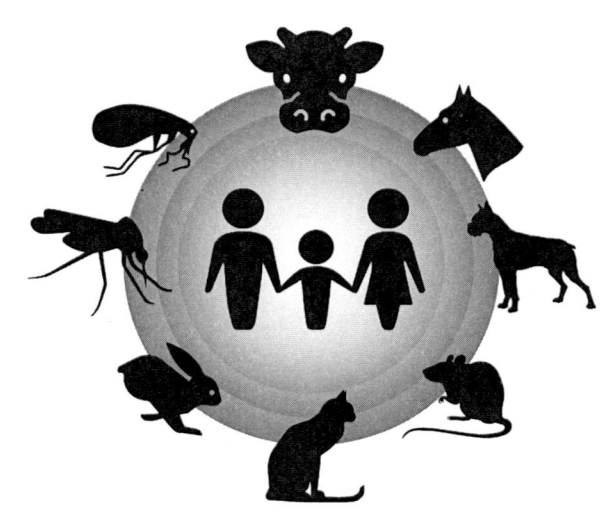

Zoonosis refers to diseases that can be passed from animals to humans.

In 2016, the world faced the growing spread of a debilitating virus called "Zika". Over 15 million individuals have already been infected by the virus. Scientists had originally thought that the virus only impacted the brains of developing fetuses and did not believe an infection posed serious problems for adults. A new study suggests that Zika also infects the brain cells of adults, causing long term memory damage.

---

[93] Every year, Salmonella causes one million food borne illnesses in the United States, with 19,000 hospitalizations and 380 deaths. CDC. https://www.cdc.gov/salmonella/

[94] Lyme disease is the most commonly reported zoonotic illness in the United States. Ranking 6th in 2015, there were more than 35,000 reported new infections."About Lyme Disease Co-Infections". https://www.lymedisease.org/lyme-basics/co-infections/about-co-infections/

This virus is chiefly spread by the Aedes aegypti mosquito, which is common throughout tropical and subtropical North, Central and South America. While healthy individuals may be able to resist the virus, those with weakened immune systems are be at serious risk. Zika is now criss-crossing the world causing major birth defects and there is no known drug cure.[95]

Two other respiratory virus outbreaks, occurring in different parts of the world, have captured the attention of global health officials: a coronavirus in the Middle East and a bird flu virus spreading in China. Each has killed tens of millions of chickens and sickened thousands of individuals.[96]

By the way, diseases like cholera, H1N1, malaria, rabies, Dengue fever, Ebola, African schistosomiasis, river blindness, and elephantiasis are not zoonotic, even though they may be transmitted by insects or use intermediate hosts. This is because they depend on the human host for part of their life-cycle. Fortunately, most of these diseases are anaerobic and respond favorably to oxygen therapy.

If the over-use and misuse of antibiotics has been one of the chief causes for the breakdown of the immune system's ability to fight off disease, can increasing the oxygen level of the blood stream really improve the functioning of the human body?

---

[95] "Zika virus may cause long-term memory damage, similar to Alzheimer's disease". http://www.telegraph.co.uk/science/2016/08/18/zika-virus-may-cause-long-term-memory-damage-similar-to-alzheime/

[96] These flu viruses occur naturally among birds. Bird flu is very contagious among birds and can make some domesticated birds, including chickens, ducks and turkeys, very sick and will kill them. H5N1 is one of the few bird flu viruses that infects humans and it is the most deadly of those that have crossed the barrier. The H5N1 virus, currently infecting birds in Asia, has caused human illness and death. It is resistant to antiviral medications commonly used for influenza. There currently is no commercially available vaccine to protect humans against the H5N1 virus that is being spread in Asia and Europe.
http://www.who.int/mediacentre/factsheets/avian_influenza/en/

Chapter Eleven:
Oxygen and the Brain

The link between insufficient oxygen and disease has now been firmly established.
Dr. W. Spencer Way, M.D.
The Journal of the American Association of Physicians

We found a dose of oxygen...can improve performance on tasks that require great mental effort.
Andrew Scholey, Director
Human Cognitive Neuroscience
University of Northumbria in Newcastle, England

The brain is an energy-demanding organ. While it makes up only 2 percent of our body's weight, it consumes more than 25 percent of our body's need for oxygen just to create the electrical energy it needs to function.

Unfortunately, the brain is incapable of storing significant amounts of glucose, which, when combined with oxygen, creates this energy. So, as mental, physical and emotional demands increase, so too does the brain's requirement for energy. If the brain does not get the energy it requires, it simply loses its ability to properly code and process sensory information.

Each of our hundred-billion brain cells, uses oxygen to stoke the fires of consciousness. Our brain's need for oxygen is more than ten times greater than the rest of our entire body.

Our brain cells are extremely vulnerable to changes in our oxygen supply. Brain cells can start dying five minutes after they are deprived of oxygen. Because brain cells will die if the supply of blood that carries oxygen is stopped, the brain has "top priority" for blood and the oxygen carried by the red blood cells. Even if other organs need blood, the body attempts to first supply the brain with a constant flow of blood.

The brain uses oxygen in the same way other organs do. Within every cell in the brain mitochondria take up oxygen and use it to convert glucose into cellular energy (ATP). Without ATP, neurons would very quickly lose their ability to fire and the brain would shut down.

Inside the skull, our carotid arteries branch into smaller and more numerous arteries, fanning out in a fantastically intricate network of lacy capillaries. This dense network is designed to reach into every crease and corner of our brain to feed "oxygen" to as many neurons as possible.[97] Yet, inevitably, some cells will get less oxygen than others. These tend to be the cells we use the least and are also the first to die off.

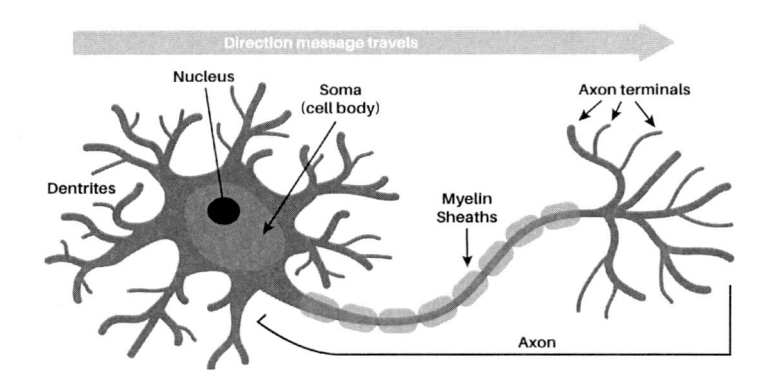

It's hard to grasp the speed that signals travel in the brain. Each neuron can shoot a signal to another neuron at more than 268 mph. The average human brain has about 100 billion neurons (or nerve cells) and many more neuroglia (or glial cells) and each one fires 5 - 50 times every second!

---

[97] Nutrients and oxygen are carried to the brain by more than 100,000 miles of blood vessels and capillaries. These vessels and capillaries are found on the surface of the brain and deep within the brain.

Neurons[98] (nerve cells) transmit signals to and from the brain at over to 268 mph. The neuron consists of a cell body (or soma) with branching dendrites (signal receivers) and a projection, which looks like a long tail,) called an axon. At the end of the axon, the axon terminals transmit the electro-chemical signal across a synapse (the gap between the axon terminal) to another neuron or a receiving cell).

A typical neuron has from 1,000 to 10,000 synapses. So, each neuron communicates with from 1,000 to as many as 10,000 other neurons, muscle cells, glands, etc. You can see how important every neuron is to our brain. Losing a single neuron can affect signals to thousands of other cells, which in turn can prevent signals to thousands more. The "chain" of memory loss can be astounding!

A one-year old baby has about 100 billion neurons and no new neurons will be formed after we reach this age. After the age of thirty, because the brain's circulatory system becomes less and less efficient, about 35,000 brain cells will die every day and 200 have died in the time it took to read this far into this book. Since we have at least 100 billion brain cells[99], this rate of loss is hardly noticeable in a single day. But the loss adds up as the years go by.

In the next week, almost a million more of our brain cells will likely die. By the time we reach 60 years old, a healthy adult will have lost more than 766,500,000 neurons. Less neurons means less memory as well as a host of other potentially serious brain disorders.

Since brain tissue cannot sustain itself without oxygen, as brain cells are depleted of oxygen, they have to convert their aerobic or oxygen-processes into anaerobic-- without oxygen—processes. This "switch" is described by Sarah Rocksworld and her research associates in "Neuro-

---

[98] The word "neuron" was created by the German scientist Heinrich Wilhelm Gottfried von Waldeyer-Hartz in 1891. He also came up with the term "chromosome".

[99] As many brain cells as there are stars in the Milky Way!

logical Research."[100] She explains that when brain cells revert to anaerobic metabolism to create energy, they lose their ability to regulate brain function. As a result, free radicals are generated that damage the brain cells.

Without oxygen, amino acids and protein parts are released that continue to damage brain cells. So, even short periods of oxygen deprivation can result in cellular death.

> "Research has shown that oxygen administration leads to improved long-term memory and reaction times compared to a control group of normal air-breathing....oxygen administration appears to facilitate cognition most effectively for tasks with a higher cognitive load."[101]

How "strong" a memory imprints in our brains depends on the strength of the synapse between the neuron cells associated with the memory. The more we practice or think about a piece of information stored in our brain, the more energy is produced and that particular synapse is stronger in imprinting the memory.

As the synapse is used more frequently, it grows in strength. This allows the memory to be more vivid and clear in our minds. But, iIf we do not access the memory very often, the synapse begins to weaken. This may cause us to forget the memory, or we will find it more difficult to remember it. None of this access can occur without an adequate supply of oxygen for neuron energy.

Increasing the amount of oxygen to the brain will accomplish two things. First, it will activate areas of our brain that are usually idle because of reduced blood oxygen nourishment. Second, providing the brain with more oxy-

---

[100] Neurological Research, March 2007.

[101] Con Stough and Andrew Scholey's (editors), "Advances in Natural Medicines, Nutraceuticals, and Neurocognition,"

gen will slow down the constant death and deterioration of our brain cells

To a serious competitive athlete, oxygen availability to the brain and muscles means the difference between peak performance or failure in competition.[102] Any athlete can attest to the fact that muscular exhaustion and mental fatigue from oxygen depletion is the primary cause for performance failure.

> "*Eventually, your muscles can no longer get enough oxygen. It's an immutable physical limit that kicks in during any sustained physical exercise and tells your body: 'This fast – but no faster.' At least, that's the theory we've been working with since 1923. But a controversial new study from researchers on three continents suggests that the famous 'VO$_2$max' – the maximum amount of oxygen that you're able to deliver to your muscles during hard exercise – isn't really a maximum at all. Your heart and lungs don't call the shots...your brain does.*"[103]

Nootropics

Is oxygen a nootropic? Nootropics, also known as "smart drugs", are cognitive enhancers. They can boost memory and help to increase focus and attention. Memo-

---

[102] Some Interesting Brain Trivia:
- If every person on the planet simultaneously made 200,000 phone calls, there would be the same total number of connections occurring as take place in a single human brain every day.
- We can retain about seven facts at any one time in short term memory, but over the long term, our brain has to forget things to make room for new memories.
- Our brain generates 25 watts of power while we are awake, enough power to illuminate a light bulb.
- Unconsciousness will occur after 8-10 seconds after loss of blood supply (oxygen) to the brain.

[103] Alex Hutchinson, The Globe (2012)

ry, as has been noted, begins to decline as early as the late teens. But there are other factors that can make memory decline faster: stress, alcohol and lack of sleep are just a few examples.

When a person learns, they require two cognitive skills: memory and concentration. Memory is the ability to remember and concentration is the power to hold our attention. Generally, nootropics consist of medications ("drugs"), dietary supplements or functional foods. Several nootropics even act as vasodilators.[104] Oxygen appears to provide a nootropic benefit[105] without the potentially adverse side effects associated with manufactured pharmaceuticals.

> *"Under the broad definition of the term nootropics is a Pandora's box of dozens of cognitive enhancing substances, including well-researched supplements like creatine, plant derivatives like L-theanine, and off label usage of the pharmaceutical modafinil (medically prescribed to treat narcolepsy). But without more oversight and long-term studies, there's really no way to know what the conse-*

---

[104] Vasodilators are medications or nutritional supplements that will open up the blood vessels.

[105] This study investigated the effect of 30% oxygen administration on verbal cognitive performance, blood oxygen saturation, and heart rate. The experiment compared normal air (21% oxygen) and hyperoxic air (30% oxygen). Accuracy rates were enhanced by 30% oxygen administration compared to 21% oxygen and blood oxygen saturation was increased significantly compared to that with 21% oxygen administration. Significant positive correlations were found between changes in oxygen saturation and cognitive performance.
The effect of transient increase in oxygen level on brain activation and verbal performance. Chung SC1, Sohn JH, Lee B, Tack GR, Yi JH, You JH, Jun JH, Sparacio R.
Int J Psychophysiol. 2006 Oct;62(1):103-8. Epub 2006 May 6.

quences of turning your brain into a chemistry experiment will be. The impact of these drugs on healthy brains – and your brain in particular — is less clear. And while it's true that a lot of healthy people take a variety of nootropics and smart drugs every day with few deal-breaking side effects, the reality is, scientists and medical professionals have no clue what the long-term impact of popping pills and stirring up powders will be on you."[106]

---

[106] The Dark Side of Smart Drugs: The dangers, risks, and side effects of nootropics. Kristen Spina. December 21, 2015
http://www.everup.com/2015/12/21/nootropics-smart-drugs-dangers-risks-side-effects/

Chapter Twelve:
Alternative Oxygen Therapies: Recharging the Immune System

Whenever the immune system deals successfully with an infection, it emerges from the experience stronger and better able to confront similar threats in the future. Our immune system develops in combat. If, at the first sign of infection, you always jump in with antibiotics, you do not give the immune system a chance to grow stronger.
Dr. Andrew Weil

Oxygen is called both a life-giver as well as a "killer." It is one of the body's primary guardians and protectors against unfriendly bacteria and other disease organisms. In fact, one of oxygen's major functions is the "disintegration" of pathogenic organisms in a process called oxidation.

Oxidation is a process where electrons are exchanged between oxygen and another atom, molecule or element creating a new molecule or atom. During this "exchange" process the donating element or molecule is changed either in its structure or its function while the oxygen atom retains its integrity.

The simplest example of oxidation is the conversion of iron (Fe^+) as it reacts with oxygen in air to form rust (iron oxide). Apples that have been cut into slices and exposed to oxygen in the air will turn brown because of oxidation. This occurs because oxygen atoms are intrinsically in need of electrons to become fully stable.

We need to remember some very basic chemistry. Every atom is surrounded by orbiting electrons. It is the number of electrons that give an atom its stability, its electrical charge ("positive" if it has extra orbiting electrons and "negative" if it is missing electrons,) and which determine the atom's ability to combine with other atoms to form more complex molecules.

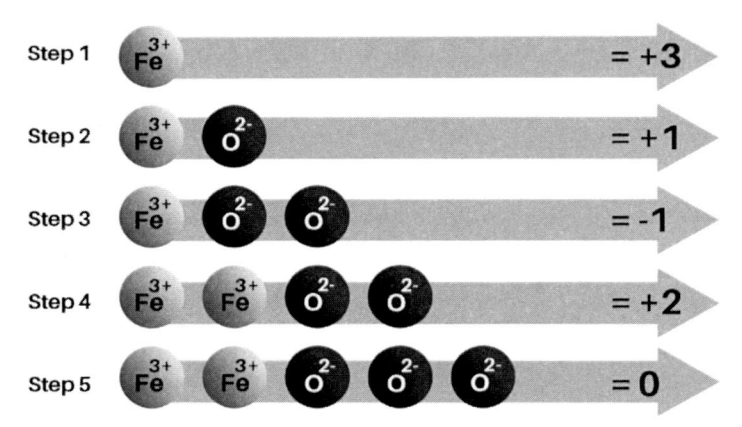

ATOMS					NET ELECTRON CHARGE
Step 1	Fe^{3+}				= +3
Step 2	Fe^{3+}	O^{2-}			= +1
Step 3	Fe^{3+}	O^{2-}	O^{2-}		= -1
Step 4	Fe^{3+} Fe^{3+}		O^{2-}	O^{2-}	= +2
Step 5	Fe^{3+} Fe^{3+}		O^{2-}	O^{2-} O^{2-}	= 0

This is an example of oxidation. The metal iron (Fe) reacts with oxygen (O) atoms to form iron oxide (Fe_2O_3) which we call "rust". In the first step, a single iron atom, which has three unpaired electrons in its outermost valence orbital shell, reacts with a single oxygen atom which is missing two electrons in its outermost shell. The combination of these atoms creates a temporary molecule Iron II Oxide (FeO) which still has one unpaired electron. Seeking stability, FeO combines with another oxygen atom which is missing two electrons creating Iron Oxide (FeO_2) which is still unstable because it is missing one electron. This molecule grabs another iron atom which creates Ferrous Oxide (Fe_2O_2). But this molecule has two extra electrons and is unstable and so grabs another oxygen atom and forms the stable molecule Ferric Oxide (Fe_2O_3) which we call rust. This is also what we call a "corrosion" action and how quickly this five step process takes place depends on temperature and water vapor.

Wisegeek.com has a great description of what an atomic orbital is:

"An atomic orbital is a region of space around the nucleus of an atom where an electron is located. The exact location can only be approximated by using the laws of probability. Atomic orbitals occupy spherical areas around the nucleus in three dimensions, so electrons do not orbit the nucleus like a planet orbits a star. There are different shapes to orbitals as well; one type that symmetrically sur-

rounds the nucleus of an atom, and another that spreads in different directions on either side of the nucleus. Each atomic orbital, no matter its type, is situated at different energy levels that extend farther from the nucleus, with the lowest energy level being the closest...There are various other shapes to atomic orbitals as well, which help to describe the nature of electrons as waves surrounding a nucleus. Atoms with a single electron are structured like a planet with an atmosphere, and atoms with many electrons seem to have a cloud of electrons surrounding them. Electrons near the nucleus have lower energies, while orbitals become more complex at higher energy levels farther from the nucleus."[107]

The strength of the attraction between atoms determines the stability of the molecules that have been created by two or more atoms. Some molecules are quite strong and resist disintegration. Others are relatively weak and break apart easily into component atomic parts or groups of atoms.

Chemical bonds are formed when the electrons in an atom interact with the electrons in another atom. This allows for the formation of more complex molecules. There are three basic types of chemical bonds between atoms: covalent, ionic and hydrogen. Covalent is the strongest bond and the hydrogen bond is the weakest.

Covalent
Bond Strength: Strong
Description: These strong bonds form when two atoms share electrons.

---

[107] Copyright © 2003 - 2013 Conjecture Corporation
http://www.google.com/imgres?imgurl=http://images.wisegeek.com/atom-vector

Example: Bonding that takes place between Oxygen and Hydrogen in water (H_2O), hydrogen gas (H_2) and the oxygen we breathe (O_2).

Ionic
Bond Strength: Moderate
Description: Oppositely charged ions are attracted to each other.
Example: The bonding between sodium (Na^+) and chloride (Cl^-) in salt (NaCl).

Hydrogen
Bond Strength: Weak
Description: Occurs in molecules that have covalent bonds. Sometimes the electrons are not equally shared; one atom tends to have an electron more often than the other atom. In this situation one atom of the molecule becomes partly negative and the other then becomes partly positive.
Example: The weak bonds between water molecules are known as "clusters" of water molecules and they form and break up constantly. another molecule example is hydrogen peroxide. it is the combination of two hydrogen atoms and two oxygen atoms (H_2O_2). In the presence of heat, sunlight (ultraviolet rays,) or when in the presence of anything acidic, hydrogen peroxide's atoms break apart to release a singlet oxygen atom (O_1) leaving the three remaining atoms to form the very strong and stable water molecule (H_2O). The singlet oxygen atom is highly unstable and needs a electron to reach a stable state. It is in this state that this single molecule will grab electrons from any other atom or molecule in its vicinity.

The Human body contains both beneficial as well as harmful microbes. Beneficial microbes, like the ones that inhabit the intestinal tract and aid in the digestive process, like acidophilus and beneficial E-coli, thrive in an oxygen-rich environment. These organisms are called "aerobic" or air-tolerant. The molecules that make up their cellular walls have very strong bonds.

However, pathogenic organisms can only exist and can only reproduce in a reduced or non-oxygen environment. These organisms are called "anaerobic" or non-air tolerant. Luckily for us, anaerobic (non-air/oxygen tolerant) unicellular bacteria, yeasts, parasites, viruses, molds, and fungi are excellent electron donors. The molecules that make up their cellular walls have very weak bonds and are easily oxidized by oxygen's need for electrons.

The current research clearly indicates that, regardless of the genetic make-up of an anaerobic organism, whenever these microbes are subjected to the presence of oxygen, these organisms self-destruct (remember what was described in an earlier chapter.)

One explanation of oxygen's "mode of action" is that oxygen, (in its various configurations, i.e. O_1, O_2, O_3, O_4. etc.,) interferes and disrupts a pathogenic organism's cytoplasmic membrane. Oxygen's oxidizing action appears to prevent the uptake of amino acids while at the same time disorganizes this membrane. This action creates a tear in the membrane structure which allows the organism's low molecular weight cellular contents to leak out. It is this cellular cytoplasmic breach that actually destroys the organism.

Oxygen, therefore, is naturally selective in what it kills. Unlike drugs and antibiotics which may kill both beneficial and disease organisms in the body, oxygen kills only harmful anaerobic organisms while allowing beneficial organisms to thrive, thus insuring good health. In addition, as was previously discussed, oxygen is the key ingredient to healthy cellular metabolism.

There is no other single atom as versatile and as crucial to our existence than oxygen. Oxygen truly is, as Dr. Stephen Levine stated, "the spark of life."[108] Given oxygen's powerful restorative and antimicrobial properties, it can come as no surprise that a number of therapeutic protocols and theories have been developed by both the traditional medical and alternative medical professions.

Before looking briefly at these therapies, it's important to remember that the immune system is the primary defense against disease, and its warriors are the white blood cells, which have already been described.

All white blood cells, especially the ones called phagocytes, destroy bacteria, dead tissue cells, protozoa, various dust particles, pigments, and other minute foreign bodies that inhabit our blood stream. The process they use depends on oxygen and is called "phagocytosis" (from the Greek, meaning "a hollow vessel that devours".)

In a remarkable process, the human body receives signals from chemicals released from bacteria and other pathogens that draws phagocytes to the area of infection. At the same time, these same substances trigger the bone marrow by telling it to manufacture and release more white blood cells to assist in the battle.

As mentioned earlier in the book, there are two main types of phagocytes called microphages and macrophages. The microphages only live for a few days and are constantly circulating in the blood stream. Fortunately, the bone marrow has a large reserve of these soldiers. These macrophages, though there are not as many of them, live longer. Unlike the microphages which wander through the body waiting to go into action, the macrophages are critically stationed throughout the body

---

[108] Op. Cit. Levine and Kidd, "Antioxidant Adaptation and Immunity, Cancer, Oxygen, and Candida Albicans".

in places that are not usually well defended by the microphages. These sites include the alveoli of the lungs, the abdominal (peritoneal) and chest (pleural) cavities, under the top layer of the skin and in the intestines.

The primary process that microphages and macrophages use to kill and digest pathogens (phagocytosis) is similar to how a unicellular amoeba gets its food, by engulfing it. The major difference is that white blood cells digest these invaders using bursts of oxygen free radicals, called "oxidative" or "respiratory" bursts, that literally tear the pathogens apart. Without these "oxygen bullets" we would not be able to withstand the invaders in our bodies.

Unfortunately, space does not permit an in-depth study of the history and the diversity of alternative oxygen therapies available today. For those with an appetite for detail, I do recommend the well documented book by journalist Ed McCabe called "Oxygen Therapies: A New Way of Approaching Disease"[109] or the short book by Dr. Kurt Donsbach called "Oxygen - Oxygen - Oxygen."[110]

In general, the term "oxygen therapies" refers to any process that increases the available oxygen in the blood stream, or any regimen that enhances the body's ability to utilize, retain or promote oxygen absorption. These therapies can be as simple as breathing exercises or can be much more complex, involving nutritional and therapeutic approaches developed and used successfully over the last 50 or so years.

Nathaniel Altman, author of the book "Oxygen Healing Therapies", presents an excellent definition of oxygen therapy and how this therapy works:

---

[109] McCabe, Ed. Oxygen Therapies: A New Way of Approaching Diseases. Energy Publications, Morrisville, NY (1994).

[110] Donsbach, Kurt, N.D., Ph.D. Oxygen - Oxygen - Oxygen Rockland Corporation: 1993.

"Oxygen therapies enhance the body's immune system and are therefore used in treating a great variety of illnesses. More than fifty diseases have been treated with oxygen therapy by doctors in the U.S. including candida, cancer, dermatitis, gynecological infections, diabetes, HIV-related problems, asthma and the Epstein-Barr virus. The effects of oxygen therapies are twofold. First, they increase the level of oxygen compounds used by the immune system to fight illness...Second, oxygen therapies increase the delivery of oxygen to the cells and therefore promote cellular respiration, which is fundamental to all life processes."[111]

Here are just a few of the more widely accepted oxygen-based therapies:

Breathing or Inhalation Therapies:

Breathing exercises are designed to utilize a greater amount of lung surface area to transfer more oxygen to the blood stream as well as to remove more carbon dioxide from the blood stream. It is believed that the average person uses only about 50% of the lungs' capacity. Therefore, deeper breathing exercises should theoretically increase blood oxygen saturation.[112]

---

[111] Altman, Nathaniel. "Bio-Oxidative Therapy". Natural Health, November/December 1995: 44.

[112] "Oxygen levels play a critical role in determining the severity of the inflammatory response and ultimately the effectiveness of anti-inflammatory drugs...Starved of oxygen the body will become ill, and if this persists we will die. The clinical application of O_2 to wounds, tumors, leukemia, and to all chronic and acute situations gets to the heart of what is right or wrong inside of us."
Anti-Inflammatory Oxygen Therapy, Dr Sircus, Ac., OMD, DM (P), Director International Medical Veritas Association and Doctor of Oriental and Pastoral Medicine, March 24, 2014. http://drsircus.com/medicine/anti-inflammatory-oxygen-therapy/

Medical Grade Oxygen:

For those with more serious bronchial or respiratory problems, bottled pure oxygen therapies may be prescribed by a medical practitioner. Pure 100% oxygen gas is very toxic to the lungs because of its oxidative potential. Therefore oxygen administered using this therapy is usually reduced in concentration to no more than 20% of pure oxygen, which approximates the oxygen content in normal air.

Nutritional Therapies:

Research has shown that a number of vitamins, minerals, amino acids and enzymes play an important role in the creation of, and use of, oxygen in the body's normal metabolic cycle. One of the body's most important and abundant enzymes is superoxide dismutase (S.O.D.) and is found in every cell in the body. S.O.D. fights harmful free radicals and turns them first, along with the enzyme catalase, into stable oxygen and hydrogen peroxide and then finally into oxygen and water. Low levels of S.O.D. increases free radical damage to the body and decreases oxygen availability.[113]

Co-enzyme Ql0 (CoQl0) is found in every cell and is essential in the transfer of electrons from one atom or one molecule to another. The human body cannot function

---

[113] When delicate SOD molecules are coupled with a protective protein derived from wheat and other plants, they can be delivered intact to the intestines and absorbed into the bloodstream, thus effectively enhancing the body's own primary defense system. Once in circulation in the bloodstream, these powerful antioxidants go to work detoxifying potentially harmful substances and reducing oxidative stress that might otherwise contribute to aging and crippling diseases such as atherosclerosis, stroke, and arthritis. By strengthening the body's primary antioxidant systems, novel SOD-boosting supplements may offer the most powerful free radical protection available today.
Dale Kiefer. "Superoxide Dismutase: Boosting the Body's Primary Antioxidant Defense". June 2006
http://www.lifeextension.com/magazine/2006/6/report_sod/Page-01

without an adequate supply of CoQl0. In fact, this enzyme has been described as the "spark" that ignites the oxygen in the cells which, in turn, reacts with glucose to create A.T.P. fuel energy. Thus, CoQl0 regulates the oxygen supply to the mitochondria as part of this energy producing cycle.

Germanium is a trace mineral that is crucial for balancing the oxygen content of the cells and helping to regulate the cell's bio-electricity. Germanium, in regulating oxygen levels, enhances the immune system. This mineral also helps remove toxic minerals from the body including mercury, cadmium and lead.

Iron, of course, is the most important mineral involved in transferring oxygen to every cell in the body. Iron forms the crucial part of the heme molecule in our red blood cells.[114] In a perfect reaction, a diatomic oxygen molecule (O_2) combines with the iron-rich heme molecule. But this attachment only remains strong until the blood cell approaches a cell that contains carbon dioxide (CO_2) as a metabolic waste product. When this occurs, the two molecules (O_2 and CO_2) exchange places.

A deficiency of iron in the body (called "anemia") results in poor body oxygen and an increase in a number of diseases. Women are particularly subject to iron deficiencies due to menstruation.

While iron supplementation is extremely important, it is important to understand that elemental iron cannot provide any nutritional support. All iron, to be biologically "active", must be consumed in a chelated form. When iron, or other minerals, are bound to an amino acid, known as a chelate, they can be absorbed more easily.[115]

---

[114] Remember, there are over 100 trillion red blood cells each containing iron in our bodies at any one time.

[115] Some chelated minerals include ferrous 'iron' gluconate, calcium gluconate, magnesium citrate, chromium polynicotinate. You can usually tell by the "ate" suffix if a mineral has been chelated.

Ginseng is a root that has been used for over 4,000 years to help build endurance and alertness. Recently, research has indicated that ginseng actually helps increase oxygen levels in the blood as well as enhances pulmonary (breathing) activity.

Ginkgo biloba is an ancient, long-living tree whose leaves yield flavonglycosides which are powerful free-radical scavengers and tissue/cell membrane stabilizers. Ginkgo strengthens and improves oxygen circulation.

Ginger is another botanical that promotes blood and oxygen circulation that also provides over 12 natural antioxidants more powerful than Vitamin E.

Magnesium oxide (MgO_2) is a remarkable mineral oxide that delivers substantial amounts of oxygen when potentiated by stomach acid or citric acid. As far back as the late 1800s, formulations containing magnesium oxide were used as a therapy and promoted by Dr. EM. Eugene Blass, a medical doctor and a professor of chemistry, histology and physiology.[116]

---

[116] Dr. Blass is considered to be one of the "fathers" of oxygen therapies. His original products, called Magozone, Calzone, Malcazone and Homozone (released in 1898), have been used to deliver cleansing and healing oxygen to millions individuals all over the world.

Chapter Thirteen
Hydrogen Peroxide Oxygen Therapy

It has been clinically demonstrated that the spread or metastasis of cancer is inversely proportional to the amount of oxygen around the cancer cells. The more oxygen, the slower the cancer spreads. The less oxygen, the faster the cancer spreads. If cancer cells get enough oxygen, they will die (cancer cells are anaerobic). It is thought that hydrogen peroxide kills cancer cells because cancer cells do not have the mechanism to break down hydrogen peroxide that healthy cells have.
R. Webster Kehr[117]
Independent Cancer Research Foundation

When it comes to hydrogen peroxide therapy there seems to be only two points of view. Supporters consider it one of the greatest healing miracles of all time. Those opposed feel its ingestion is exceptionally dangerous, and only the foolhardy could think of engaging in such behavior.[118]
Dr. David G. Williams, M.D.

More than 6,000 articles have been published in the medical journals about the benefits of hydrogen peroxide (H_2O_2) therapies during the last 70 years.[119] Most of these articles focus on the disinfecting and healing properties of

---

[117] Robert Webster Kehr, For more tan 15 years, Mr. Kehr has published information about natural cancer treatments since the founding of his Independent Cancer Research Foundation. https://www.cancertutor.com

[118] Original title: Hydrogen Peroxide - Curse or Cure?, Posted July 17, 2003 http://educate-yourself.o...genperozide17jul03.shtml

[119] During this same period it is estimated that hydrogen peroxide therapy has been administered by an estimated 15,000 European doctors, naturopaths and homeopaths to more than 10 million patients.
Madison Cavanaugh. The One-Minute Cure: The Secret to Healing Virtually All Diseases. Think-Outside-the-Book Publishing, Inc. August 21, 2008.

this remarkable molecule which easily breaks down into water (H_2O) and oxygen (O_1). It is the release of the singlet oxygen atom (O_1) that may provide benefit to the body.

$$H_2O_2 + = H_2O + O$$

When hydrogen peroxide (H_2O_2) is exposed to sunlight or heat, a chemical reaction occurs. The molecule is split apart and reforms into two new molecules: water (H_2O) and singlet oxygen (O).

Hydrogen peroxide is actually manufactured by the body as an instrumental part of the our first line of defense against invading pathogens. The release of an oxygen atom, which occurs when hydrogen peroxide meets a pathogen in the blood stream, deactivates the cellular integrity of that pathogen as I described in an earlier chapter.

As was previously explained, the manufacturing or "creation" of hydrogen peroxide is one of the primary functions of the white blood cells. However, the body also acquires hydrogen peroxide in a number of healthy foods including fruits and some vegetables. Hydrogen peroxide is also a key ingredient in colostrum, the first milk that babies drink from their mothers' breasts.

Traditional hydrogen peroxide therapies include the consumption of diluted food-grade hydrogen peroxide, intravenous drips and injections of a highly diluted solution. It is important to understand that food-grade hydrogen peroxide is very different than the hydrogen peroxide that can be purchased at the supermarket or drug store. Food grade hydrogen peroxide usually contains 25% to 35% hydrogen peroxide while general-use hydrogen peroxide is only three percent strength. The general-use peroxide solution also contains small amounts of the chemical acetanilide (C_8H_9NO) which is used as a stabilizing agent. Acetanilide is toxic and the ingestion of even small amounts of it affects the central nervous system, can cause irritation and exposure can lead to dermatitis. Never ingest non-food grade hydrogen peroxide.

Remember that hydrogen peroxide is not a stable molecule. In its concentrated form, it is highly corrosive and can cause severe burns and destroy tissues. It can also become highly flammable. Lastly, the FDA has issued warnings about using and consuming food grade hydrogen peroxide.[120]

From an atomic perspective, hydrogen peroxide (H_2O_2) is composed of four atoms, two each of both oxygen and hydrogen. Because this molecule is electrically unstable,

---

[120] Then again, the FDA has also issued warnings about using many natural alternative therapies. Here's what the FDA has posted on their website about hydrogen peroxide therapies:

"FDA Warns Consumers Against Drinking High-Strength Hydrogen Peroxide for Medicinal Use: Ingestion Can Lead to Serious Health Risks and Death." The U.S. Food and Drug Administration (FDA) is warning consumers not to purchase or to use high-strength hydrogen peroxide products, including a product marketed as '35 Percent Food Grade Hydrogen Peroxide,' for medicinal purposes because they can cause serious harm or death when ingested. FDA recommends that consumers who are currently using high-strength hydrogen peroxide stop immediately and consult their health care provider. FDA is working to stop companies selling high-strength hydrogen peroxide from making illegal medical claims about their products. These claims are illegal because these products do not have FDA approval and are therefore being sold illegally for medical indications without any proven clinical value. The products can instead cause significant harm…Ingesting hydrogen peroxide can cause gastrointestinal irritation or ulceration. Intravenous (IV) administration of hydrogen peroxide can cause inflammation of the blood vessel at the injection site, gas embolisms (bubbles in blood vessels), and potentially life-threatening allergic reactions. FDA previously warned consumers, in an April 1989 press release, about the illegal promotion of industrial-strength hydrogen peroxide to treat AIDS and cancer, following at least one related death in Texas and several injuries requiring hospitalization."
http://www.fda.gov/NewsEvents/Newsroom/PressAnnouncements/2006/ucm108701.htm

the second oxygen atom is easily coaxed from the molecule, which then becomes two separate molecules: a water molecule (H_2O) and a singlet oxygen molecule (O_1). This change in physical configuration when the molecule encounters ultraviolet light, heat or when it contacts organic matter.

The singlet oxygen molecule is a strong oxidizing agent. O_1 seeks electrical stability since it needs an additional electron so the electron orbits can settle into a more stable state. One of the places it can get an electron is from an anaerobic micro-organism or even from a healthy cell.

As was discussed in a previous chapter, oxygen atoms oxidize single cell organisms. The loss of electrons disorganizes their basic electrical cellular structures and functions and so they die. Visualize someone sticking a finger into an electrical socket and receiving a shock. That is what happens to a microorganism when it comes into contact with oxygen.

The primary factor driving the growth in hydrogen peroxide consumption world-wide today is the concern for the environment. Hydrogen peroxide naturally decomposes into two safe ingredients, water and oxygen. This makes hydrogen peroxide an excellent disinfectant as well as a bleaching agent replacement for other very toxic oxidizing compounds, like chlorine.

Until the early 1980s, hydrogen peroxide demand was equally distributed among the wood pulp bleaching, chemical synthesis, disinfectant and the textile bleaching industries. Today, pulp bleaching accounts for over 67% of the demand for hydrogen peroxide in the U.S. and Canada and 48% of Western Europe's demand.[121] The rapid

---

[121] Six companies dominate the hydrogen peroxide marketplace. They are, FMC Corporation (U.S.A, Degussa AG (Germany), DuPont (U.S.A), Oxysynthese S.A (France), and Mitsubishi Gas Chemical Company, Inc. (Japan). A sixth, Solvay, now claims that it is the largest supplier of stabilized hydrogen peroxide for the cosmetic and food industries in the U.S.)

growth for just this application alone has been driven by consumer pollution awareness and tighter governmental pollution regulations.

There are a number of "grades" of hydrogen peroxide based on the concentration of oxygen-based molecules in each grade. These grades run from a low of three percent to a high of over 90%. They are:

1. 3% H_2O_2 which is used primarily for topical disinfecting. (This is the typical drug store variety.) This grade contains four or more toxic stabilizers to help reduce the molecular breakdown of the molecule and to prevent the premature release of oxygen. This grade is made using 50% super peroxide which is diluted to a three percent level.
2. 6% H_2O_2: This is used primarily by beauticians for the topical beaching of hair. It is available in a number of strengths and also contains toxic stabilizers.
3. 30% Reagent H_2O_2: This grade is primarily used for medical research, though it also contains toxic stabilizers.
4. 30% - 32% Electronic Grade H_2O_2: This grade is used by the electronics' industry to wash transistors and integrated chips before assembly and contains toxic stabilizers.
5. 35% Technical Grade H_2O_2: This grade is used for a variety of scientific and industrial applications. This grade contains trace amounts of phosphorus and is used to counter-balance dissolved chlorine in water. This grade is not intended for human consumption.
6. 35% Food Grade H_2O_2: This grade is used for a variety of applications in the food preparation, food manufacturing and food packing industries, especially for cheese, whey and egg products. This grade is still very caustic and in this high concentration it can easily burn the skin. 35% food grade hydrogen peroxide

must be diluted in order for it to be safe to handle, use and consume. Remember that even though the F.D.A. has indicated that hydrogen peroxide is neither toxic nor carcinogenic, the F.D.A. strictly forbids the use of H_2O_2 for oxygen therapy usage.
7. 90% H_2O_2: This grade is used by N.A.S.A. as a fuel propellant oxygen source for the space program. This grade is extremely combustible and dangerous.

As you can see, the only hydrogen peroxide grade that can be used for human consumption is a dilution of the 35% food grade solution. To be "safe", this grade must be diluted with water by at least 98% to prevent cellular oxidative damage.

Hydrogen peroxide oxygen therapies have been used for over 150 years with varying degrees of success. However, now that new and safer stabilized oxygen technologies exist, these newer oxygen therapy technologies appear to be more preferable. More importantly, these new products do not require toxic stabilizers to insure that the molecules do not break down and prematurely release the oxygen.

Cosmetics and dental products, including tooth pastes, mouth washes, and gels, that claim they contain stabilized hydrogen peroxide, may contain industrial or medical grade H_2O_2 that also contain toxic stabilizers. Putting this grade of peroxide on the skin or in the mouth, in any concentration, may actually be harming the body rather than bringing the body the added benefits of oxygenation. If the label does not state that food grade hydrogen peroxide is being used in its diluted form, then it would probably be advisable to refrain from using the product(s) until the actual contents are determined.

As part of an alternative therapy, H_2O_2 is a double edged sword. While it may indeed help oxygenate the blood, bringing countless benefits and relief from various diseases and ailments, it does have a darker side that can produce dangerous side effects. Many articles and books on the subject of H_2O_2 oxygen therapies fail to mention that extreme caution should be used whenever using peroxides for medicinal or preventative alternative therapies. In every case, individuals should consult with a qualified medical practitioner who has experience in a variety of oxygen therapies before personally using hydrogen peroxide for any protocol or to self-administer treatments for any ailment or condition.

Perhaps the insight and admonition of Dr. Cordel Logan, N.D., award-winning author of the book Medicine at the Crossroads, should be considered whenever administering hydrogen peroxide therapies. He wrote:

> *"Certainly excess hydrogen peroxide is harmful (may even aggravate Candida, cause rectal bleeding, and damage the digestive system) ... Excessive hydrogen peroxide may inactivate adenylate cyclase (forms cyclic AMP), and cytochrome P-450 (a microsomal enzyme). It may inactivate SOD, rhodanese, trypsin, kinases, and other enzymes. Hydrogen peroxide inhibits immunoglobulins and causes red blood cell lysis (bursting)...Chromosomal damage has been reported. Dimethyl sulfoxide (DMSO), a scavenger for hydroxyl radicals, does not react with hydrogen peroxide or superoxide thus is not protective here ... Extra hydrogen peroxide may combine with superoxide to form the hydroxyl radical which is a highly reactive free radical. This can cause peroxidation of unsaturated fatty acids. The healthy electrical charge from sialic acid can disappear leading to premature aging and other degenerative problems."*[122]

---

[122] Logan, Cordell, Ph.D., N.D. Medicine at the Crossroads, Logan Press, Logan, UT (1993)

As with many nutritional and alternative medicine approaches to health, too much of a "good thing" can be detrimental. Hydrogen peroxide, for nearly two centuries, has provided numerous health benefits. Caution, wisdom, and discernment as to the best approach to using H_2O_2 therapies should be the only approach to take.

Chapter Fourteen:
Ozone Therapies

Ozone therapy can do what no drug on the planet can do. It can reactivate and regenerate cells that have been previously unable to efficiently metabolize oxygen. Ozone therapy improves the flexibility and elasticity of the blood vessels, thereby increasing blood supply and life giving oxygen to the heart and vital tissue. Ozone also oxidizes fatty substances like plaque that adheres to arterial walls and helps normalize cholesterol and triglycerides. Ozone, when correctly administered, has no side effects.
Dr. Robert H. Sorge, N.D, Ph.D, PND[123]

Ozone is a gas molecule containing three oxygen atoms (O_3) joined together by a weak electrical bond. It is present in the atmosphere, and its blue color is what gives the sky its wonderful hues.

The ozone molecule is unstable. It quickly breaks apart into a diatomic oxygen molecule (O_2) and a singlet oxygen molecule (O_1) in approximately 30-40 minutes after it has been created.

As far back as 1785, scientists noted ozone's distinctive odor and disinfecting properties. It was not until 1840 that ozone got its "name" from the Greek "ozein" which means "odorant".

Ozone has not only been "officially" used as treatment for many wounds[124], it is now used extensively to purify water in residential and commercial pools and in waste water

---

[123] Dr. Robert H. Sorge, N.D., Ph.D., PND. Dr. Sorge attended The United States School of Naturopathy and Applied Sciences, the oldest Naturopathic School in the country, organized in 1898. In 1972, Dr. Sorge received his Doctorate of Philosophy in Naturopathic Medicine. In 2001, Dr. Sorge received his (PND), Philosopher of Naturopathic Medicine, the highest degree given by this institution and only seven degrees awarded by the school in 110 years of its history.

[124] One of the earliest mentions of ozone therapy in the U.S. dates back to 1885 when The Florida Medical Association published the article "Ozone" by Dr. Charles J. Kenworthy, M.D., Jacksonville, Florida.

treatment plants around the world. Because ozone breaks down into harmless oxygen molecules, it is the ideal replacement for carcinogenic chlorine in these applications. However, in numerous countries in the world, other than the United States, ozone has been used as a blood treatment to kill viruses and to increase blood oxygenation.

Studies of ozone "blown" over wounds show a dramatic improvement in the healing of those wounds as well as a significant reduction in infections. Burns particularly respond well to ozone treatments.[125]

Ozone is 10 times more soluble in water than atmospheric oxygen (O_2) and may be bubbled in bath water to help treat and disinfect the skin for eczema and skin ulcers. It can also be added to drinking water to help increase blood oxygen levels, though the water needs to be immediately consumed since ozone decomposes so quickly into its oxygen parts (O_2 and O_1).

Ozone does have its medical drawbacks. The singlet oxygen molecule is highly reactive oxidative atom. If not used or administered properly, ozone can "burn" the skin or organs. If inhaled in large quantities, ozone can also be toxic. Ozone should never be administered for any alternative therapy situation unless under the supervision of a medical practitioner.

The use of ozone therapy in the U.S. has had considerable resistance from the intrenched pharmaceutical and traditional medical communities. Their efforts are supported by ongoing attacks by the FDA. Here's what was published in Natural News that explains the main "legal" issues:

> *"In Germany, ozone therapy has been widely used since 1959. There have been 10,000 German doctors using ozone therapy for close to 10 million patients for various diseases with a 90 percent cure*

---

[125] See Appendix 5 for a very brief outline of the use of ozone for medical purposes over the last 150 years.

rate and virtually no side effects. Yet the FDA disregards this as 'anecdotal evidence', while the pharmaceuticals with 'scientific evidence' kill many and cure few. Russia claims 40 years of successful ozone therapy, especially for tuberculosis. A medical report from Russia claims that those who are cured do not have a reoccurrence. Cuba authorized ozone therapy in 1986 and uses it in all its hospitals. So if you can get to Cuba, you may get a good deal! But there are ozone clinics in Mexico and other parts of the Caribbean as well. In the 1960's, Robert Atkins, MD of Atkins Diet fame, temporarily lost his license after it was discovered he had cured, repeat cured, a woman's breast cancer by injecting the tumor with O_3. He used his NYC weekly radio show to announce exactly what had happened. The resultant public outcry forced the NY State Medical Board to reinstate his license, but with Atkins' agreement to quit using or publicizing ozone therapy. The FDA suppresses ozone therapy in every way possible. Prior to the 1940's, it was commonly used in the USA. The first USA ozone generator was created in 1896. Successful ozone therapy in America dates back to that time, before the FDA was created."[126]

Ozone therapy is an accepted and recognized procedure in Bulgaria, Cuba, the Czech Republic, France, Germany, Israel, Italy, Mexico, Romania and Russia. It is currently used legally in 16 nations. Eleven states in the USA, (Alaska, Colorado, Georgia, Minnesota, New York, Ohio, Oklahoma, Oregon, South Carolina and Washington,) have already passed access-type bills to ensure that alternative

---

[126] Fassa, Paul. "The FDA Continues to Suppress Ozone Therapy Despite Proven Efficacy", naturalnews.com, Friday, February 19, 2010. http://www.naturalnews.com/028201_ozone_therapy_FDA.html#ixzz2VjRZW9jT

therapies are available to consumers[127]. Efforts are also underway in California Delaware, Florida, Kentucky, New Jersey, Massachusetts, Missouri and Kentucky to pass similar legislation.

> *"One study evaluating the adverse side effects of over 5 million medically administered ozone treatments found that the rate of adverse side effects was only 0.0007 per application. This figure is lower than any other type of medical therapy."*[128]

---

[127] There are numerous ways to administer ozone. They include: Intravenous Injections, Hyperbaric Major Autohemotherapy, Ozonated Saline IV, Direct Ozone IV (DIV), RHP (Recirculatory Hemoperfusion), EBOO (Extracorporeal Blood Oxygenation and Ozonation), Intraairticular Injections (Prolozone), Intramuscular Injection, Subcutaneous Injection, Intradermal Injection, Insufflations, Ozonated Water and Ozone Sauna
From: "WHAT IS OZONE THERAPY?"
http://thepowerofozone.com/all-about-ozone/what-is-ozone-therapy/

[128] Altman, Nathaniel. The Oxygen Prescription: The Miracle of Oxidative Therapies. Healing Arts Press, Rochester, VT. 2007

Chapter Fifteen:
Hyperbaric Oxygen Therapies

I've seen partially paralyzed people half carried into the HBOT chamber, and they walk out after the first treatment. If we got to these people quickly, we could prevent a great deal of damage.
Dr. Edgar End, M.D.
Clinical Professor of Environmental Medicine
Medical College of Wisconsin[129]

It has taken almost a hundred years for Western medicine to accept the healing benefits of hyperbaric oxygen therapy (HBOT). Today, even the world renowned Mayo Clinic now provides oxygen therapy to its patients and the hospital describes the process this way:

"Hyperbaric oxygen therapy involves breathing pure oxygen in a pressurized room. Hyperbaric oxygen therapy is a well-established treatment for decompression sickness, a hazard of scuba diving. Other conditions treated with hyperbaric oxygen therapy include serious infections, bubbles of air in your blood vessels, and wounds that won't heal as a result of diabetes or radiation injury."[130]

The first notable use of oxygen as a therapy was promoted by Dr. Orval J. Cunningham in 1918. Dr. Cunningham used a chamber he constructed to treat victims of the

---

[129] December 1, 1937 was a momentous day in the history of diving. Not only was a new world record set at 420 feet but it was also the first significant use of a helium-oxygen breathing mixture in an open water environment outside the confines of a dry hyperbaric facility. Dr Edgar End, M.D., of the Marquette University School of Medicine in Milwaukee, WI, was the person responsible for calculating the helium-oxygen breathing mixtures and the decompression schedule used for the world record dive.

[130] May Clinic Online. http://www.mayoclinic.com/health/hyperbaric-oxygen-therapy/my00829

Spanish influenza epidemic that swept across the USA during the closing days of the First World War.[131] The chamber he built was eight feet diameter by 30 feet long. Because he had excellent results with patients suffering from pneumonia and the flu, he was encouraged enough to build additional chambers.

In the late 1920s, Dr. Cunningham built the world's largest functional hyperbaric chamber in Cleveland, Ohio. It was a 64 foot steel sphere "hyperbaric medical hotel" with five floors of living space including a restaurant. Unfortunately, the Great Depression in the 1930's ended his project and the giant chamber was scrapped for the war effort in the 1940s.

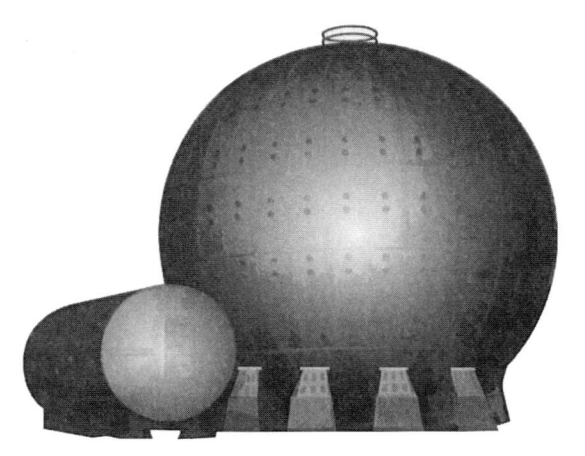

The Cunningham hyperbaric medical hotel c1930 was more than 64 feet in diameter and was five floors of living space and restaurants.

Dr. Cunningham treated diseases such as syphilis, hypertension, diabetes mellitus, and cancer. His reasoning was based on the assumption that anaerobic infections

---

[131] Jacobson JH and others. "The Historical Perspective of Hyperbaric Therapy". Annals of the New York Academy. of Sciences 117:651, 1965.

play a role in the "etiology"[132] of all such diseases. Yet, for many decades afterwards, hyperbaric oxygen therapy (HBOT) chambers were used only to treat decompression sickness and air embolisms experience by divers and aviators.

During the early 1960s, HBOT was proposed as a treatment for cancer, heart attacks, senility and other conditions. The medical profession and the pharmaceutical industry, as a whole, discounted its use and its benefits.

Dr. Izaak F. A. van Elk, M.D., a cardiologist, was one of the very brave medical professionals to challenge the status quo. His research, and his successful effort to construct the first therapeutic hyperbaric oxygen chamber in the U.S.A., was completed at Lutheran General Hospital, Park Ridge, Illinois in the early 1960s.

Dr. van Elk's hope was that the oxygen therapy would help cure patients suffering from the physiological after-affects of heart attacks (specifically coronary occlusions). He and his team also tried the chamber on patients suffering from strokes and dementia.[133]

In 1962, Doctors Smith and Sharp reported the enormous benefits of HBOT in treating patients suffering from carbon monoxide poisoning.[134] Their research rekindled international interest in the benefits of the therapy, and HBOT was relaunched into the modern medical arena.

Hyperbaric units were rapidly constructed at Duke University, New York Mount Sinai Hospital, Presbyterian Hospital and Edgeworth Hospital in Chicago, Good Samaritan in Los Angeles, St. Barnaby Hospital in New Jersey, Harvard Children's Hospital, and St. Luke's Hospital in Milwaukee.

---

[132] The cause, set of causes, or manner of causation of a disease or medical condition.

[133] http://wiki.answers.com/Q/Who_invented_hyperbaric_oxygen_therapy

[134] Smith G., Sharp G. R. Treatment of carbon monoxide poisoning with oxygen under pressure. Lancet 1960;1:905–906.

Chambers were were also built at numerous international sites.[135]

HBOT involves the inhalation of oxygen rich air under a pressure greater than one atmosphere[136]. This increased atmospheric pressure helps deliver more oxygen to the tissues and to the cells to enhance healing as well as to improve the immune system's ability to fight off infection.

Medical research has confirmed that HBOT provides varying benefits for decompression sickness, carbon monoxide poisoning, acute tissue damage, burns, headaches, strokes, head injuries, autism, post traumatic stress disorders and bacterial and viral infections.[137]

While some of the mechanisms of action of HBOT, as they apply to healing and reversal of symptoms, are yet to be discovered, it is known that HBOT:

- greatly increases oxygen concentration in all body tissues, even with reduced or blocked blood flow;
- stimulates the growth of new blood vessels to locations with reduced circulation, improving blood flow to areas with arterial blockage;
- causes a rebound arterial dilation after HBOT, resulting in an increased blood vessel diameter greater than when therapy began, improving blood flow to compromised organs;
- stimulates an adaptive increase in superoxide dismutase (SOD), one of the body's principal, internally

---

[135] Smith G, Sharp GR. Treatment of coal gas poisoning with oxygen at two atmospheres pressure. Lancet 1:816, 1962.

[136] "Atmosphere" is the pressure exerted by the earth's atmosphere at any given location. In measurement, it is the equivalent to the pressure exerted by a column of mercury 29.92 inches (760 mm) high, or 1013 millibars (101.3 kilopascals). Sea level is usually considered as "one atmosphere" of pressure.

[137] There have been reports indicating that the Ebola (flesh eating) virus was controlled in a number of victims that were fortunate enough to undergo HBOT treatments.

produced antioxidants and free radical scavengers; and,
- aids the treatment of infection by enhancing white blood cell action and potentiating germ-killing antibiotics.

Yet, despite over a century of use in medical settings, HBOT still remains a controversial therapy among the medical community. Even so, there are now more than 500 HBOT centers in cities and hospitals all across America and Canada. and hundreds more in Europe and throughout the rest of the world.[138]

As Dr. Jeffrey A. Niezgoda, MD wrote in a recent article:

"The overall acceptance and validation of hyperbaric medicine as a true medical specialty is probably the biggest change that has happened over the last 5 to 10 years. When I was doing my fellowship we had to really work for patient referrals. There were a lot of naysayers. There was a lot of skepticism. We were criticized for the lack of hyperbaric literature. We worked hard to convince our colleagues that HBO was a valid adjunctive treatment. It often felt like I had to be a cheerleader or salesman for this treatment modality. Fortunately for our patients, much of this has changed. Some really excellent clinical and research studies with supporting publications have appeared in the literature. Based on the literature and excellent clinical out-

---

[138] Two excellent books that go into much more detail about this very affordable and often successful treatment process are:
Harch M.D. Paul G. and McCullough, Virginia. The Oxygen Revolution: Hyperbaric Oxygen Therapy: The New Treatment for Post Traumatic Stress Disorder (PTSD), Traumatic Brain Injury, Stroke, Autism and More. Hatherleigh Press, 2010
Neubauer, Richard A. and Walker, Dr. Morton. Hyperbaric Oxygen Therapy, Avery Trade, 2001.

comes, hyperbaric has truly emerged as a primary advanced treatment modality for wound care patients. Younger doctors appear more ready to accept case studies which highlight some really amazing success stories and refer their patients for care. I think mainstream medicine has finally accepted hyperbaric as a viable treatment. It is rewarding after all these years of hard work, advocating for a treatment that I believe in based on outstanding results and limb salvage, to have physicians who had previously doubted and questioned hyperbaric—the plastic surgeons, the vascular surgeons, the general surgeons—now calling and asking for our help."[139]

---

[139] Dr. Jeffrey A. Niezgoda, MD, FACHM, MAPWCA is the current President of the American College of Hyperbaric Medicine (ACHM). He is also the Medical Director, at The Center for Comprehensive Wound Care and Hyperbaric Oxygen Therapy, St. Luke's Medical Center, Aurora Health Care, Milwaukee, Wisconsin, U.S.A.
Hyperbaric Oxygen Therapy News, August 6, 2012
http://hyperbariclink.blogspot.com/

Chapter Sixteen:
Oxygenated Bottled Water

Filthy water cannot be washed.
WEST AFRICAN PROVERB

Water is life's mater and matrix, mother and medium. There is no life without water.
Albert Szent-Gyorgyi
Hungarian Biochemist
1937 Nobel Prize for Medicine

All the water that will ever be is, right now.
National Geographic
October 1993

Tap water quality is one of the most pressing health threats to residents of the U.S. and around the world today. Each year the correlations between contaminated drinking water and cancer, learning disabilities, and asthma are becoming stronger and clearer. Even if tap water has gone through municipal treatment before reaching our home faucet, it is often far from safe.

In many cases, municipal water treatment facilities actually add dangerous chemicals to water in the process of treatment. Municipal water treatment methods are often old and outdated; consequently, they are simply incapable of dealing with the dangerous assortment of contaminants that may be present in drinking water. And, in spite of government regulations of drinking water by the EPA and FDA, dangerous contaminants are still present in drinking water.

While the EPA sets maximum contaminant levels (MCLs) for a broad range of drinking water contaminants, these levels are not at "zero", where they should be for our safety. As a result, chemicals and pollutants are present in our tap water, even if the EPA claims they are in small amounts.

Many people may say that attacks on the quality of tap water (potable water) are simply scare tactics designed to increase profits for bottled water and water treatment companies. But, the large increases in the number of individuals suffering from cancer and other diseases does bear a causal relationship to the poor quality of drinking water.

Based on research conducted by the World Health Organization (WHO), here are the top ten countries in the world with the best drinking water, from the best to worst:

Switzerland	Italy
Norway	United Kingdom
Luxembourg	Sweden
France	Germany
Austria	New Zealand

Note that the United States is not even listed in the top ten. In fact the U.S. ranks as sixty-fourth in the world for the quality of its drinking water.

What follows is a brief explanation of contaminants that are very likely in our tap water as well as a discussion of how these contaminants may affect our health, body oxygen levels and how they depress the immune system.

Chlorine is perhaps one of the most dangerous and insidious poisons in our drinking water supply. Surprisingly, it is a normal municipal additive to drinking water. Water treatment facilities use chlorine as a powerful disinfectant to kill or inactivate biological water contaminants. But that same chlorine, which is so toxic to biological contaminants, is also poisonous to our bodies. Chlorine in drinking water is currently the leading cause of bladder and rectal cancer and asthma. Health officials are now linking chlorine ingestion to breast cancer. Chlorine also robs the body of precious oxygen as they body attempts to detoxify and eliminate this poison.

Lead makes its way into tap water through corrosion of the pipes in a home's plumbing system. Many of the old water conduit systems in large cities may also contain lead pipes and fittings. Because lead contamination occurs after municipal treatment, there is no way that municipal facilities can control for it.

In the United States, 310,000 children under five years old have unsafe levels of lead in their blood. Minute levels of lead can cause headaches, stomach pain, behavioral problems and anemia (where not enough healthy red blood cells can deliver oxygen to the brain and other cells). Lead in drinking water is especially harmful for pregnant mothers because its presence is directly linked to severe developmental delays and/or learning disorders in children.[140]

Every year, nearly one billion pounds of pesticides are sprayed onto fields and orchards around the country. "Pesticide" is a general term for substances that are used to poison or control weeds, insects, molds, rodents, etc. The pesticides most acutely dangerous to man are insecticides and rodenticides, although pound for pound, herbicides are the most widely used type of pesticide.

Pesticides enter surface and ground water primarily as runoff from crops and are most prevalent in agricultural areas. Pesticides are also used on golf courses, forested areas, along roadsides, and in suburban and urban landscape areas.

Since World War II, herbicide and insecticide applications to crops have grown enormously and have contaminated almost every groundwater supply in the United States. Approximately half of the U.S. population obtains its drinking water from groundwater sources and as much as

---

[140] The E.P.A. permits lead levels in drinking water to be less than 15 ppb however there is absolutely no safe level for lead exposure.

97% of the population in agricultural areas use groundwater as the primary source of drinking water.[141]

Pesticide use has grown because not only must our own expanding population be supplied with more food, but also demand for our food has dramatically increased from other countries around the world. The United States is the largest producer of food products in the world, due a great deal to our agri-technology and the use of modern pesticides to control the insects, weeds, and other organisms that attack food crops.

Just one example of a dangerous pesticide is methyl iodide. It is chemical that has been directly linked to cancer and late-term miscarriages and, because it's a gas, it easily drifts miles from fields and into nearby communities.

Methyl iodide was approved for use as a pesticide in the early 2000s over the objection of more than 50 eminent scientists, among them six Nobel laureates in chemistry. Though methyl iodide is used primarily on strawberries, it is also registered for use on tomatoes, peppers, for nurseries and on soil prior to replanting orchards and vineyards. Dr. Kathleen Collins, Ph.D., a cancer cell specialist at the University of California at Berkley, stated:

> *"Methyl iodide causes late term miscarriages, contaminates groundwater and is so reliably carcinogenic that it's used to create cancer cells in labora-*

---

[141] For many years, people believed that the soil and sediment layers deposited above an aquifer acted as a natural filter that kept many unnatural pollutants from the surface from infiltrating down to groundwater. By the 1970s, however, it became widely understood that those soil layers often did not adequately protect aquifers. Despite this realization, a significant amount of contamination already had been released to the nation's soil and groundwater. Scientists have since realized that once an aquifer becomes polluted, it may become unusable for decades, and is often impossible to clean up quickly and inexpensively.

http://www.waterencyclopedia.com/Oc-Po/Pollution-of-Groundwater.html#ixzz4RoV3ghl1

tories. It is included in California's Proposition 65 list of chemicals known to cause cancer. The pesticide poses the most direct risks to farm workers and neighboring communities because of the large quantities that would be applied to fields and its tendency to drift off site through the air. Use of methyl iodide is anticipated to be similar to methyl bromide and could top 6-10 million pounds a year in California alone."[142]

Pharmaceuticals[143], which include antibiotics, hormones, mood stabilizers, and other drugs, are also present in trace amounts in our drinking water supplies and even in some brands of poorly filtered bottled water. In one investigation, the details of which were reported by the Associated Press, drinking water supplies in 24 major metropolitan areas were found to include drugs.[144]

---

[142] Kathleen Collins, Department of Cellular Biology. UC Berkeley. http://www.collective-evolution.com/2016/07/26/chilling-testimony-from-a-cancer-cell-specialist-makes-one-thing-utterly-obvious-about-our-food/

[143] A vast array of pharmaceuticals including antibiotics, anti-convulsants, mood stabilizers and sex hormones have been found in the drinking water supplies of at least 41 million Americans, an Associated Press investigation shows. To be sure, the concentrations of these pharmaceuticals are tiny, measured in quantities of parts per billion (ppb) or trillion (ppt), far below the levels of a medical dose. Also, utilities insist their water is safe. But the presence of so many prescription drugs and over-the-counter medicines like acetaminophen and ibuprofen in so much of our drinking water is heightening worries among scientists of long-term consequences to human health.

"Pharmaceuticals found in drinking water, affecting wildlife and maybe humans". Jeff Donn, Martha Mendoza and Justin Pritchard, Associated Press Writers.
http://hosted.ap.org/specials/interactives/pharmawater_site/day1_01.html

[144] Doheny, Kathleen. "Drugs in Our Drinking Water? Experts put potential risks in perspective after a report that drugs are in the water supply." http://www.webmd.com/a-to-z-guides/features/drugs-in-our-drinking-water

Most of us do not realize that more than ten percent of the water we drink is actually recirculated from sewage treatment plants. This water finds its way back into ground water sources. Because we flush pharmaceuticals down the drain, and these chemicals are excreted in our urine, it is almost impossible to prevent them from contaminating municipal and well water sources. Sewage treatment plants are simply not equipped to eliminate them during processing nor are municipal water plants capable of filtering them out either. As Kathleen Doheney writes for WebMed:

> *"Although levels are low -- reportedly measured in parts per billion or trillion -- and utility companies contend the water is safe, experts from private organizations and the government say they can't say for sure whether the levels of drugs in drinking water are low enough to discount harmful health effects. 'Low levels of pharmaceuticals in the water supply have been a concern for a decade or longer', says Sarah Janssen, MD, PHD, MPH, a science fellow at the Natural Resources Defense Council, an environmental action group. 'Ever since the late 1990s, the science community has recognized that pharmaceuticals, especially oral contraceptives, are found in sewage water and are potentially contaminating drinking water.'"*[145]

The parasites Giardia and Cryptosporidium have been the plague of the water treatment industry for decades. Resistant to chlorine, these protozoa can lead to severe and widespread outbreaks of gastrointestinal diseases if released into a municipal water system. They often make their way into tap water because of sanitation system

---

[145] Ibid.

breakdowns, and municipal water treatment facilities have no fail-safe way to control them.[146]

> "There are many causes of tap water contamination, ranging from agricultural runoff, to improper use of household chemicals, and everything in between. Few of us realize the extent or impact of these low level synthetic chemicals in the water we use. While the standard use in our society of over 80,000 different synthetic chemicals has offered added convenience and productivity to our lives, it has also come at a tremendous price...Our use of man-made chemicals has become so extreme that we can now find traces of these low level SOCs (synthetic organic chemicals) in virtually every public water supply around the world. A recent report by the Ralph Nader Study Group, after reviewing over 10,000 documents acquired through the Freedom Of Information Act, confirmed, 'U.S. drinking water contains more than 2,100 toxic chemicals...'"[147]

Of course, bottled water is nothing more than reconstituted, rebottled tap water. We know that water treatment facilities cannot completely remove chlorine and other dangerous contaminants, drugs, chemicals and microorganisms from drinking water. All of these wreak havoc on our immune systems and organs, especially the liver and brain. Toxins force the body to accelerate an immune response depleting oxygen reserves and reducing the

---

[146] To view one of the best videos to date on water quality issues, and a winner of more than a half dozen international awards, please visit the "FLOW" website. The New York Times wrote about the movie: "An astonishingly wide-ranging film. An informed and heartfelt examination of the tug of war between public health and private interests."
http://www.flowthefilm.com/

[147] Ralph Nader Research Institute
http://www.pureeffectfilters.com/2100-chemicals-in-drinking-water

amount of oxygen necessary for normal healthy metabolism.

We have already learned that increased air pollution, consuming processed and refined foods, a lack of exercise and stress rob oxygen from the body. Now add all of the other toxins, chemicals and hormones in our drinking water and you have a formula for a health disaster.

Is it really then any wonder why immune-related diseases are on the increase? Is it a surprise when microorganisms and diseases we once thought were eradicated or under control are on the rise again? So, is it even possible to make water healthier by adding oxygen to it before we drink it?

The idea of adding additional oxygen to water is, of course, nothing new. In 1840, Schonbein[148] discovered ozone (O_3), bubbled it through water and quantified its properties. Almost 50 years later, in 1886, the ability of ozone to disinfect polluted water was recognized throughout Europe. Between 1891 and 1906, Germany, the Netherlands and France commission the first municipal ozone plants for drinking water.

By 1915, at least 49 major ozonated water installations were on line throughout Europe. It took almost seventy additional years, until 1982, for the USFDA to establish and adopt GRAS (generally regarded as safe) declarations for ozone use in municipal and bottled water. In 1987, the City of Los Angeles' water ozonation plant went on line after seven years of testing.

We know that ozone is an unstable yet highly beneficial molecule. It is the triatomic form of oxygen. Instead of the normal arrangement of two atoms of oxygen (O_2), ozone is comprised of three atoms of oxygen (O_3). Ozone, however, does not want to stay in that triatomic state very long and

---

[148] Christian Friedrich Schönbein (18 October 1799 – 29 August 1868) was a German-Swiss chemist who is best known for inventing the fuel cell (1838) and his discoveries of guncotton and ozone.

will rapidly break down from O_3 to $O_2 + O_1$ typically within 20 minutes after O_3 has been formed. O_1 (the "singlet" oxygen atom) is highly reactive. It is missing one electron and will take one from any another atom or molecule that will donate one.

Water Source	Amount of Dissolved O_2
Ocean	4 - 11 mg/L (p.p.m.)
Running Stream or River	5 - 14 mg/L (p.p.m.)
Pond	0 - 8 mg/L (p.p.m.)
Lake	2 - 11 mg/L (p.p.m.)
Bottled Water	0 - 5 (p.p.m.)
Tap Water	5 - 6 (p.p.m.)

The amount of oxygen (O_2) that can be dissolved in water depends on the temperature as well as the source of the water. the higher the amount of oxygen in water, the more healthy the water is for consumption.

Ozone, therefore, is not the ideal "oxygenator" for use in bottled water because it is unstable. It is used more appropriately as a disinfectant or to assist in decomposing other toxic ingredients that may be in water.

Unlike ozone, which is unstable, diatomic oxygen (O_2) is a more stable molecule of oxygen and has been injected as a gas in bottled water -- just like carbon dioxide (CO_2) is used in carbonated beverages before the bottle is sealed. In addition, just like CO_2, O_2 will also escape when the cap is opened.

O_2 oxygen molecules are very small (about 292 pm[149]) and are able to move easily through the spaces between

---

[149] A picometer (symbol "pm") is a unit of length in the metric system, equal to one trillionth (i.e., 1/1,000,000,000,000) of a meter. It can be written in scientific notation as 1×10^{-12}.

plastic water bottle molecules. Multi-layered plastic bottles can reduce this migration process, but these bottles are also impregnated with oxygen scavenging compounds that are designed to neutralize oxygen, which further diminishes the benefits of the trapped oxygen gas in a water bottle. The shelf-life of oxygenated (O_2) bottled water can be measured in days and weeks, rather than in months.[150]

Diatomic oxygen reaches equilibrium in water at between 6-15 mg/L[151], depending on the water's temperature. The colder water is, the more dissolved oxygen it can trap and retain in solution

The only commercially viable alternative to pressurized diatomic oxygen in bottled water is to use a relatively new form of stabilized polyatomic tetraoxygen (O_4). Fortunately, in June of 2013, such a bottled water was released and is now available to consumers. The water is called OXIGEN WATER® and is exclusively sold by Formula4®.[152] This is the only oxygenated bottled water that contains stable molecules of oxygen and which has supported research to demonstrate its efficacy.

So, in the end, the noble goal of adding oxygen to water in order to make it more "healthy" has actually been achieved. It has taken nearly more than 125 years to take the healing power of oxygen from a challenged concept, to an accepted ingredient to promote health, healing and energy. And this leads us to a discussion about concentrated oxygen therapy in the form of oxygen supplements.

---

[150] LifeO2 Super Oxygenated Drink was the first commercially available oxygenated water. Released in 1998, the technology was flawed because the oxygenated water had a short shelf-life due to the fact that the oxygen gas escaped from the bottles.

[151] The measurement in "mg/L" stands for milligrams per liter. When measuring particles, atoms or molecules in water, the acronym "ppm" (parts per million) is often used These two annotations can be used interchangeably.

[152] See: https://www.drinkoxigen.com

Chapter Seventeen:
Stabilized Oxygen:
Introducing Vitamin O

> "Oxygen is needed for the body. We can be without food and water for a lengthy time. We can be without oxygen only for a few seconds...It is the spark of life."
> Dr. Charles H. Farr, M.D., Ph.D.
> O2 Therapies[153]

What distinguishes stabilized oxygen therapies from the ones described in the previous chapters is that the products in this category are considered "foods" or "dietary supplements" and are not subject to licensing by, or the approval of, the U.S. Food and Drug Administration (USFDA).

In spite of the lobbying efforts by the pharmaceutical and medical industries, a successful grassroots campaign was launched by U.S. consumers in 1994 to push the U.S. Congress into enacting legislation to protect dietary and food supplements from regulation by the FDA. The legislation was called the Dietary and Supplement Health Education Act (DSHEA), and its passage by Congress, began a brief "golden age" where it became easier for consumers to purchase supplements and for manufacturers to bring new natural remedies to market without the invasive intervention of the F.D.A.

In view of all the scientific evidence available today, it is clear that an excellent oxygen ratio in the blood stream is

---

[153] Since the late 1970s, a small group of practitioners has advocated the use of intravenous infusions of hydrogen peroxide for a multitude of indications. Their rationale is based largely on the research and clinical experiences of the late Charles H. Farr, MD, PhD (1927-1998). A true champion of this therapeutic method, Charles H. Farr is often referred to as the "Father of Oxidative Medicine." Dr. Farr discovered "a positive metabolic effect to intravenous infusions of hydrogen peroxide," and authored an impressive workbook on the subject.

a prime requirement for good health. Unlike using hydrogen peroxide and chlorine dioxide, which were the forerunners to the newer oxygen-rich liquid supplements, these oxygen formulas hold the oxygen molecules in a stable molecular configuration.

Before we take a deeper look into this nutritional category, it is time to deal with some of the incredulous things being said and written about "stabilized oxygen" from so-called medical and scientific experts.

"You have to be a fish with gills..."

Many writers, professional practitioners, medical doctors and scientists have made it their sworn duty to destroy the credibility of oxygen supplementation. They claim that only a fish with gills can benefit from stabilized oxygen, or any oxygen molecules for that matter, that become dissolved in a liquid. These individuals, trained in the ways of Western Medicine and science, really should have a stronger duty to testing their theories before stating that their beliefs are conclusive scientific fact.

As a scientist[154], the first question one should ask about oxygen oral supplements is: "Is it really possible to absorb oxygen through the digestive tract if the oxygen were dissolved in a liquid medium? Unfortunately, this is something that many medical professionals and scientists believe is

---

[154] The Scientific Method is an organized way that helps scientists answer a question or solve a problem. There are typically six steps:
1. Purpose/Question – What do you want to learn?
2. Research – Find out as much as you can that relates to the purpose/question.
3. Hypothesis – After doing the research, attempt to predict the answer to the problem.
4. Experiment – Design a test or procedure to find out if the hypothesis is correct.
5. Analysis – Record the data that describes what happened during the experiment.
6. Conclusion – Review the data and check to see if the hypothesis was correct.

completely impossible, and they have had no problem staking their reputations on this assertion, just as if it were a medical "fact". But, all scientific facts must be validated by what is called the "scientific method". Sadly, those with a predisposition of unbelief in the benefits of oxygen supplementation completely disregard their scientific roots.

In 1989, a movie was released, called "The Abyss", in which the lead actor, Ed Harris, playing the part of the underwater miner Virgil 'Bud' Brigman, puts on a special diving suit that uses a super-oxygenated liquid, instead of compressed oxygen, for deep underwater diving. Many believed that this was Hollywood science fiction. However the concept of "liquid breathing" actually began in the mid 1960s when:

> "...Dr. J. Kylstra, a physiologist at the State University of New York at Buffalo, realized that salt solutions could be saturated with oxygen at high pressures. Working in a US Navy recompression chamber, Kylstra performed an experiment to see if mice would be able to move the saline solution in and out of their lungs, while extracting enough oxygen from the fluid to be able to survive."[155]

The test animals survived for almost 18 hours, but carbon dioxide was not removed fast enough from the system and quickly built up to near-toxic levels. This had to be solved before liquid breathing could be used by humans. Why this interest in liquid rebreathing? Because liquid breathing solutions, like perfluorooctyl bromide (also called

---

[155] Gresh, Lois H. and Weinberg, Robert. The Science of Superheroes. John Wiley & Sons, Inc., Somerset, NJ. 2003. pp. 60-61.

perflubron[156]) have been found to be useful as either blood substitutes or may be delivered directly into the lungs of patients suffering from acute respiratory failure, infections, severe burns, or who have inhaled toxic substances. "Once inside the lungs, perflubron enables collapsed alveoli to open and permits a more efficient transport of oxygen and carbon dioxide."[157]

In 1966 Dr. Leland Clark, M.D. and Dr. Golan, M.D. also experimented with liquid breathing, testing their theories on anesthetized mice. They knew that oxygen and carbon dioxide are very soluble in fluorocarbon liquids like freon. Dr. Clark proposed that, if the alveoli of the lungs can draw oxygen out of the liquid and unload carbon dioxide back into the liquid, these fluorocarbons could support the respiration of animals. Testing his theory, he discovered that indeed the theory was valid.[158]

Dr. Corrine Leach, M.D. of State University (Children's Hospital) of New York (SUNY), based on this earlier research, has treated dozens of premature infants with partial PFC liquid ventilation therapy, between 24 to 76 hours after birth, without difficulties or any adverse side effects. While some of the infants died of complications, unrelated to the liquid ventilation, others survived. A study, based on

---

[156] Perflubron (PFC) is clear, colorless, odorless, nonconducting, and nonflammable. It is approximately twice as dense as water, and is capable of dissolving large amounts of physiologically important gases, mainly oxygen and carbon dioxide. PFCs are chemically stable compounds and are not metabolized in body tissues.
Haeberle, Helene A., Nesti, Frances, Dieterich, Hans-Juergen, Gatalica, Zoran and Garofalo, Roberto P. "Perflubron Reduces Lung Inflammation in Respiratory Syncytial Virus Infection by Inhibiting Chemokine Expression and Nuclear Factor–κB Activation", American Journal of Respiratory and Critical Care Medicine, Vol. 165, No. 10 (2002), pp. 1433-1438.

[157] Op. cit. Gresh and Weinberg.

[158] Clark Jr., Leland C. and Gollan, Frank. "Survival of Mammals Breathing Organic Liquids Equilibrated with Oxygen at Atmospheric Pressure". Science 24 June 1966: Vol. 152 (#3730) Pages 1655-1802.

her applications was completed and published in 2002 in the New England Journal of Medicine and she concluded:

> "Partial liquid ventilation leads to clinical improvement and survival in some infants with severe respiratory distress syndrome who are not predicted to survive."[159]

Of course, we are not fish and our bodies were not designed with gills that can pull oxygen out of water. However, our bodies are remarkably resilient enough that oxygen, present in high enough concentrations in a liquid medium, can indeed be directly absorbed by the lungs into the blood stream.

Given established physiological research, this same dissolved oxygen, in a liquid medium, should indeed also be absorbed through the digestive tract. This diffusion action is no more of a surprise than the absorption of oxygen through the lungs.

Can, from a biological perspective, dissolved gasses, like oxygen, can be absorbed into the body at any point in, and at any time during, the digestive process? We do know that the digestive process begins in the mouth (oral cavity) and ends at the colon. In one of the most widely used and highly acclaimed medical textbooks on physiology, Dr. Arthur Guyton, M.D. and John E. Hall, Ph.D., agree that gas absorption does indeed occur through the digestive tract.[160]

All molecules and ions in the body's fluids, including water and dissolved gasses in water, are in constant motion,

---

[159] Leach, M.D., Corrine, "Partial Liquid Ventilation with Perflubron In Premature Infants with Severe Respiratory Distress Syndrome". The New England Journal of Medicine, Volume 335, September 12, 1996, Number 11. pp. 761-767.

[160] Guyton, Arthur C. The Textbook of Medical Physiology, (5th Edition.) Pennsylvania: WB Saunders Co., 1976.

which is called "diffusion". It is through simple diffusion that these molecules move through the intermolecular spaces and through the lipid layers of the cells' membrane openings. Drs. Guyton and Hall wrote:

> *"One of the most important factors that determines how rapidly a substance will move through the lipid bilayer is the lipid solubility of the substance. For instance, the lipid solubilities of oxygen, nitrogen, carbon dioxide, and alcohols are high, so that all these can dissolve directly in the lipid bilayer and diffuse through the cell membrane in the same manner that diffusion occurs in a watery solution...Especially large amounts of oxygen can be transported in this way: therefore oxygen is delivered to the interior of the cell almost as though the cell membrane did not exist."* The author's go on: *"The rapidity with which water molecules can penetrate most cell membranes is astounding."*[161]

Since water can easily pass in and out of the cells, does this water also contain oxygen? Does water passing through the gastrointestinal tract also penetrate the tract's wall barriers so that the body absorbs it? Dr. Guyton confirms that this is exactly the case. He describes the digestive process whereby carbohydrates, fats and proteins, as well as water, electrolytes and gasses, like oxygen, are indeed absorbed in the digestive tract.[162]

Dr. Guyton makes the important point that a great deal of water is absorbed into the body during the digestive process every day. In fact, this quantity can be as much as nine liters (nearly two and one half gallons) of water a day. The stomach is a poor absorptive area and he points out that "only a few highly lipid-soluble substances, such as al-

---

[161] Ibid.

[162] Ibid.

cohol, gasses (O_2 and CO_2) and some drugs, like aspirin, can be absorbed in small quantities."[163]

Whatever amount of oxygen is not absorbed through the stomach lining passes with the water that travels through the digestive tract into the small intestine. Every day, the small intestines absorb about eight liters (over two gallons) of water. The small intestine's absorption capacity is actually greater than this and is capable of absorbing up to as much as 20 liters of water (over five gallons) every day.

As oxygenated water passes into the large intestines, additional water and ions are absorbed, as much as an additional seven liters. Therefore, the potential for absorption of water throughout the digestive system is extremely high, up to a maximum potential of nearly 27 liters (over seven gallons) of water every day.

Is it not obvious that the oxygen in stabilized oxygen solutions may be easily absorbed, along with all the other components found in water, into the body? It should be no surprise then that some of these oxygen molecules will find their way into the blood stream. To believe that this cannot take place is simply ignoring the facts. It is like believing the world is flat and you will fall off sailing to the edge without getting in a boat and testing your convictions. While, at the same time, you condemn anyone who disagrees with you.

In correspondence with researcher and physiologist Dr. Neil Fleming, Ph.D.[164], I had the opportunity to ask for his educated opinion on this specific issue. Here are excerpts of what he wrote to me:

> "***Humans don't need gills to breathe:*** *Most skeptics point to the lungs as the primary argument for dismissing the concept of oxygen ingestion. It is*

---

[163] Ibid.

[164] Dr. Neil Fleming, Ph.D., Human Performance Laboratory, Anatomy Department, Trinity College, Dublin, Ireland

true that (under most circumstances) blood leaving the lungs is almost maximally saturated with oxygen. Therefore any tiny amount of oxygen which enters the blood via ingestion would be rendered useless once the blood passes through the lungs. This may well be the case for all systemic tissues downstream of the lungs. However, skeptics ignore one key location where ingested oxygen may be of significant benefit; the liver.

All blood perfusing the GI-tract must first pass through the liver before it can be returned to the right side of the heart and pumped back to the lungs. The liver is one of the most metabolically active organs in the body. It is the primary site of metabolism for a number of nutrients including alcohol, glucose and lactate. In addition, liver cells are extremely sensitive to changes in O_2 concentration, such that a small increase in oxygen results in a large increase in metabolic activity. It is therefore possible that ingested oxygen could influence liver metabolic rate.

"**There is no evidence that oxygen can be ingested:** *Several animal studies have reported that oxygen is absorbed through the GI-Tract. These invasive studies in cats and rabbits observed significantly higher O_2 concentrations in the hepatic portal vein. While these studies have not been replicated in humans, the results demonstrate that the process of absorbing O_2 from the gastro-intestinal tract is at the very least possible and arguably plausible in humans.*

"**Even if we could ingest a small amount of oxygen, it would have no effect:** *It is true that most studies examining oxygenated water report no ergogenic effects. However, the vast majority of these studies are not looking in the right place. Several studies have reported no change in either maximal or sub-maximal oxygen consumption as measured by indirect calorimetry. These studies are inherently flawed, since indirect calorimetry is based* on the Haldane Transformation. This equation assumes O_2 consumption is equal to the difference between inspired and expired O_2. It therefore does not take into account potential O_2 ingested. Regardless, it is highly unlikely that a small amount of O_2 ingested would have any effect on whole body systemic oxygen consumption or oxygen saturation, since all blood leaving the lungs is already maximally saturated with O_2. However, several studies have reported lower lactate concentrations during and after exercise. Other studies have reported faster clearance of alcohol. These findings would suggest that liver metabolism is up-regulated following ingestion of oxygenated water."

Chlorine Dioxide and Hydrogen Peroxide Oxygen Supplements

It is important to state that no chlorine dioxide oxygen supplement is approved for human consumption by the FDA even though many have been marketed and sold in this manner.[165] The oxygen atoms in these formulas are chemically bonded to chlorine salts, like sodium chloride (NaCl), which is common table salt. The combination of oxygen, chlorine and sodium atoms forms a chlorine dioxide molecule, which is also called "sodium chlorite" (NaClO_2).[166]

In order for the body to access the O_2 molecule, bound together in a sodium chlorite molecule, this molecule must be torn apart. The belief is that stomach acid (hydrochloric acid or HCl) is what releases the oxygen atoms in this molecule so that this oxygen, in theory, is absorbed into the

---

[165] Under 21CFR178.1010, the FDA has approved the use of chlorine dioxide only as a disinfectant for water treatment and to clean uncut and unpeeled produce.

[166] Coincidentally, common household bleach contains one extra hydrogen atom and is called "sodium hypo-chloride", or NaHClO$_2$, making it almost identical to sodium chlorite.

blood stream through the stomach and intestinal linings. The decomposition of the chlorite molecule must be quite rapid for the absorption to be effective.

Unfortunately, there is really no quantitative evidence, or even credible research, that demonstrates that chlorite does release its oxygen as O_2 in the stomach so that it can be dissolved into the blood stream. However, it is entirely possible that it does. But because no research has ever been conducted, we just do not know how much oxygen actually gets into the blood stream and what positive physiological affect it may have on the body.

The first mention of a chlorite-based stabilized oxygen supplement has been attributed to a solution developed by Dr. William F. Koch, M.D., Ph.D. There are a few anecdotal comments that indicate that one version of his formula was used at some point by N.A.S.A. for the space research program, though this has never been confirmed. Whether true or not, chlorine dioxide liquid solutions, like those used by Dr. Koch, would certainly have been ideal for astronauts to use in space to destroy bacteria and viruses.[167]

Hydrogen peroxide (H_2O_2) has also been called a stabilized oxygen supplement, but because of its instability, it really is not one. Food grade hydrogen peroxide has been used in various formulations for more than 100 years. While it is true that the oxygen atoms of hydrogen peroxide have been "bound" to the hydrogen atoms to form a quasi-stabilized molecule, hydrogen peroxide is not stable. It just cannot be compared fairly to the traditional oxychlorine nutritional supplements on the market today.

Dr. John Muntz, D.O., Ph.D., a noted nutritional research scientist, summarized the value of stabilized oxygen in an article in Health World. He wrote:

---

[167] McCabe, Ed. Oxygen Therapies: A New Way of Approaching Diseases. Energy Publications, Morrisville, NY (1994).

"Combine a poor diet with a lack of proper aerobic exercise (low oxygen intake), stress, alcohol and cigarettes, and there are compelling reasons to believe that many of us may be oxygen deficient. Can we then improve matters? The answer is obviously -- yes. We can improve our diet, take proper exercise, give up the things that are clearly harmful. But to change our lifestyles or avoid stress may not be so easy to achieve. It is in this context perhaps, that the case for oxygen supplementation is strongest. Stabilized oxygen...has been described as the vital nutrient -- vitamin 'O'. But can you simple take it as a daily oxygen supplement? Once again, the answer is yes...What then is the downside? There is none...The major constituents and by products have been tested extensively throughout the world without any detrimental effects on humans at the recommended levels. Controversy does exist -- but it is not about the value of oxygen or the safety of stabilized oxygen. The controversy surrounds the micro-biochemical mechanisms that operate at the cellular level, i.e. do the results stem from improved cellular efficiency, through detoxification, better intra-cellular energy transfer systems, enhanced cellular metabolic efficiency, or some of these, or all of these? Whatever the answer, if the downside is zero the potential upside is so great that the case for 'vitamin O' as a supplement for our oxygen needs is a very strong one indeed."[168]

Vitamin "O", the oxygen nutrient, was first given its name by Dr. Stephen Levine, Ph.D. when he called it the "very spark of life!"[169] The belief is that stabilized oxygen supplements are packed with nutrient oxygen which is why

---

[168] Muntz, John, D.O., Ph.D. 'The Case for Stabilized Oxygen". Health World, August 1991: 12.

[169] Op. cit. Levine and Kidd. "Antioxidant Adaptation and Immunity, Cancer, Oxygen, and Candida Albicans"

it continues to be called, by many scientists and writers, like Dr. Levine, Vitamin "O".

While Vitamin "O" is not really a vitamin, oxygen certainly fits the definition of a vitamin: a substance found in foods, (or the environment) that is necessary for life, but not necessarily manufactured by the body.

Since oxygen alternative approaches to health have been used effectively by health care professionals and documented in over 5,000 published articles during the last 100 years. The published research and articles indicate that a number of physiological factors rob oxygen from our bodies. Some of these have been mentioned previously, but here is the list:

Toxic Stress

Whether as a result from the water we drink, the air we breathe or the food we eat, our bodies are bombarded daily by chemical cocktails containing some 75,000 different toxic contaminants, hormones and pharmaceuticals, most of which did not exist twenty years ago. Oxygen is essential for the body to metabolize and eliminate these chemicals. Here's what one research scientist wrote:

> *"Recent studies of our level of knowledge of chemicals' toxicity and impacts on public health and the environment demonstrate that we know very little about most industrial chemicals and pesticides in commercial use today. We are flying blind. Despite our lack of information about these substances, every day government agencies and others make decisions permitting their use and release into the workplace and environment based on the belief of an acceptable risk and a minimal impact. We are generally deciding that these substances are innocent until proven guilty. There are at least 75,000 chemicals in commerce today. Roughly 1,000 new chemicals are put on the market each year. Almost*

> none of the 75,000 chemicals have been adequately analyzed for their full impact on the environment and human health, and most have not even received basic toxicological testing."[170]

The alarm about the long-term toxicity to the human body from these virtually untested and quickly approved chemicals has been the concern of physiologists for more than three decades. As more and more chemicals are introduced, the result is multiplying the toxicity of each chemical on its own.

> 'Scientific studies have found that exposure to multiple chemicals can have additive or synergistic effects in humans, and a few recent studies have begun to assess these combined effects. Studies have indicated that combinations of chemicals – for example the plasticizer diethyl hexyl phthalate widely used in vinyl products combined with other common toxicants (e.g., the solvent trichloroethylene or the pesticide heptachlor) – are much more powerful, and potentially damaging, than single chemicals alone Long-term exposure to multiple chemicals can have cumulative effects and may affect the susceptibility of humans to diseases in ways that are not well-understood. In addition, virtually nothing is known about the cumulative impacts of chemicals combined with other stressors such as diet, poverty, physical stress, etc.'[171]

---

[170] Estabrook, Ph.D., Tom and Tickner, Sc.D., "Facing Our Toxic Ignorance" Massachusetts Precautionary Principle Project.
http://sustainableproduction.org/precaution/back.brie.faci.html

[171] Narotsky, M. et.al. 1995. "Non-additive developmental toxicity in mixtures of trichloroethylene, di(2-ethylhexyl) phthalate and heptachlor in a 5x5x5 design," Fundamental and Applied Toxicology, 27: 203-216; E.J. Ritter et.al. 1987. "Teratogenicity of di(2-ethylhexyl) phthalate, 2-ethylhexanol, 2-ethylhexanoic acid, and valproic acid, and potentiation by caffeine," Teratology, 35: 41-46.

Emotional Stress

Adrenaline and adrenaline-related hormones are created by the body during emotionally stressful times. In the last 30 years, the level of daily stress has increased dramatically. The body must use its available oxygen to metabolize these chemicals back out of the body to reestablish metabolic balance. Research confirms that stress has not only increased but that illnesses related to stress have a long-term impact on our health and on society as well.[172]

Stress is not just an epidemic in the United States, it is a global problem. Take a moment to complete this basic stress test. Read the statements that follow and if you answer "yes" to three or more of these stress indicators, then you are living a stress-filled life. Are you:

- Experiencing disrupted sleep patterns?
- Getting less than 5 hours sleep a night?
- Feeling overwhelmed and drained by day-to-day activities?
- Experiencing mood swings?
- Getting angry or upset easily with family members or colleagues at work?
- Having memory loss and concentration issues?
- Distracted at work or with family demands?
- Experiencing headaches, sore eyes, tension in the shoulders and neck?
- Over-eating, binging or snacking on junk foods?
- Finding you have no appetite at all?
- Lacking the motivation to exercise?
- Experiencing more body aches and pains, digestive issues and mid-life problems?

---

[172] Stress symptoms affect our bodies, our thoughts and feelings, and our behaviors. Stress that is left unaddressed and resolved can be a contributing factor to high blood pressure, heart disease, obesity and diabetes. The consistent and ongoing increase in heart rate, and the elevated levels of stress hormones and blood pressure, will take a toll on the human body.

- Feeling like you want to escape away from it all and hide, that you don't want to face each day?
- Fantasizing about escaping your job, home, country, marriage, relationships, etc.?
- Feeling tired and exhausted half way through each day?[173]

The Global Association for Stress confirms that:

- *More than 80% of workers around the world feel stress on the job and nearly half say they need help in learning how to manage stress. More than 42% say their co-workers need such help as well.*
- *Workplace tress levels are rising rapidly each year with more than 60% of all workers in the major industrial countries experiencing workplace stress. China has the highest incidence of workplace stress at more than 86% of the workforce showing symptoms and stress-related disorders.*
- *For example, in Australia, more than 91% of the adult population reports experiencing stress in at least one significant area of their lives.*[174]

Dr. Robert Ader, M.D.[175], an experimental psychologist and professor of psychiatry and psychology at the University of Rochester School of Medicine and Dentistry, was the first scientist to explain how mental processes influence the

---

[173] Most people answer "yes" to three of the statements. If you answer "yes" to five or more, you are seriously stressed and this stress is having a major impact on your health and reducing available oxygen in the blood stream.

[174] Global Organization for Stress. http://www.gostress.com

[175] Dr. Robert Ader (February 20, 1932 – December 20, 2011) was an American psychologist and academic who co-founded psychoneuroimmunology, a field of study which explores the links connecting the brain, behavior, and the immune system. Dr. Ader was a professor emeritus at the University of Rochester Medical Center.

body's immune system. He called this field of medicine "psychoneuroimmunology ". His research changed modern medicine's approach to stress-related illness.

Others that followed in his footsteps include Dr. Kenneth Pelletier, M.D. He described psychoneuroimmunology as the "study of the intricate interaction of consciousness (psycho), brain and central nervous system (neuro), and body's defense against external infection and internal aberrant cell division (immunology)"[176]

Today, it is widely accepted that between 70% and 80% of all health-related problems are either precipitated by, or aggravated by, emotional, physical or psychological stress. These health problems include type II diabetes, colds, flu, migraines, lupus and cancer. In each case, a lack of oxygen at the cellular level is a functional catalyst in the rise of these disease conditions.

Physical Trauma and Infections

Bacteria and viruses exert tremendous stress on the body's immune system. Traumatic injuries also tax the body's immune system. When these situations occur, the immune system is robbed of the oxygen that is necessary for the body's normal metabolic functions.

Reduction In Available Oxygen

Studies reveal that increased environmental pollution and "green plant" destruction have affected the concentration of the amount of oxygen in our atmosphere over the last 200 years.

Many scientists believe that the oxygen content has dropped by over 50% from what it was when the dinosaurs roamed the earth. Others contend that the industrial revo-

---

[176] Pelletier. Kenneth R. and Luskin, M.D, Fred. Stress Free for Good. HarperOne, HarperCollins Publishers, New York. 2005

lution impacted the oxygen content causing it to decline by as much as three to five percent or more.

> "Professor Robert Berner of Yale University has researched oxygen levels in prehistoric times by chemically analyzing air bubbles trapped in fossilized tree amber. He suggests that humans breathed a much more oxygen-rich air 10,000 years ago. Further back, the oxygen levels were even greater. Robert Sloan has listed the percentage of oxygen in samples of dinosaur-era amber as: 28% (130m years ago), 29% (115m years ago), 35% (95m years ago), 33% (88m years ago), 35% (75m years ago), 35% (70m years ago), 35% (68m years ago), 31% (65.2m years ago), and 29% (65m years ago). Professor Ian Plimer of Adelaide University and Professor Jon Harrison of the University of Arizona concur. Like most other scientists they accept that oxygen levels in the atmosphere in prehistoric times averaged around 30% to 35%, compared to only 21% today – and that the levels are even less in densely populated, polluted city centers and industrial complexes, perhaps only 15% or lower. Much of this recent, accelerated change is down to human activity, notably the industrial revolution and the burning of fossil fuels. Professor of Geological Sciences at Notre Dame University in Indiana, J. Keith Rigby, was quoted as saying: 'In the 20th century, humanity has pumped increasing amounts of carbon dioxide into the atmosphere by burning the carbon stored in coal, petroleum and natural gas. In the process, we've also been consuming oxygen and destroying plant life – cutting down forests at an alarming rate and thereby short-circuiting the cycle's natural rebound. We're artificially slowing

down one process and speeding up another, forcing a change in the atmosphere.'"[177]

Poor Eating Habits

Consuming high amounts of unsaturated fats[178] reduce oxygen in the blood stream. Foods with high fat content and low nutrient values, like junk food and highly-processed foods, have less than half of the oxygen content than do foods containing complex carbohydrates. Even eating what we believe is healthy food lacks the bountiful vitamins and minerals that was in raw fruits and vegetables just a hundred years ago. In fact, Dr. Bernard Jensen, one of the foremost nutritionists of the 20th century, called the food we now eat "an empty harvest".[179]

Lack of Exercise

Exercising increases the body's metabolic rate as well as the intake of oxygen to help cleanse the body of built-

---

[177] "The oxygen crisis" Peter Tatchell, Guardian News and Media Limited https://www.theguardian.com/commentisfree/2008/aug/13/carbonemissions.climatechange

[178] Saturated fats are found in butter, cheese, red meat and other animal-based foods. Decades of sound science has proven that eating high amounts of these fats on a daily can raise "bad" cholesterol and puts us at a higher risk for heart disease.

[179] Jensen, Bernard and Anderson,Mark. Empty Harvest: Understanding the Link Between Our Food, Our Immunity, and Our Planet, Garden City, New York: Avery Publishing, 1990.
One of America's foremost pioneering nutritionists and authors, Dr. Bernard Jensen began his career in 1929 as a chiropractic physician. He soon turned to the art of nutrition in search of remedies for his own health problems. He observed firsthand the cultural practices of people in more than fifty-five countries, discovering important links between food and health. In 1995, I was fortunate to meet Dr. Jensen at his Hidden Valley Ranch (Escondido, California) which served as his retreat and learning center. Over the years, Dr. Jensen received a multitude of prestigious awards and honors for his work in the healing arts. These honors include Knighthood in the Order of St. John of Malta, the Dag Hammarskjold Peace Award of Belgium, and an award from Queen Juliana of the Netherlands.

up toxins. A sedentary lifestyle reduces the body's ability to process toxic contaminants and to perform normal functions while decreasing available body oxygen.

Types of Oxygen Supplements

Over the last 25 years, numerous studies have been conducted to determine the safety and efficacy of stabilized oxygen supplements. All confirm, in one degree or another, positive results.

Dr. James Berg, in his article 'Technical Discussion: Stabilized Oxygen", stated that stabilized oxygen may include O_2, or chlorine dioxide or chlorite (ClO_2).[180] Commonly used oxidants, as described by herbalist and write Brian Goulet, Certified Herbalist. These oxidants include oxides of oxygen (ClO_2, ClO, ClO_3, ClO_4, etc.), ozone (O_3) and hydrogen peroxide (H_2O_2).[181]

Best-selling author, international speaker, and one of the major authors on oxygen therapies today, Ed McCabe, wrote:

> *"The so-called stabilized oxygen products are actually salts of oxygen diluted in water. These safe as directed, yet potent oxidizers, sometimes contain various proprietary additives to enhance their effectiveness. They are essentially a formulation mixing a solution of mildly buffered sodium chlorite with deionized water. These products are usually weakly buffered to an alkaline pH of around 12% but unlike highly buffered drain cleaners or other strong alkaline solutions, they immediately lose their alkalinity upon contact with any substance that is of lower pH. Bacteria, viruses, the acid mantle of human*

---

[180] Berg, Dr. James D., Ph.D. 'Technical Discussion: Stabilized Oxygen". Search For Health (U.S.A.), 1988.

[181] Goulet, Brian. "Confessions of an Herbalist: The Magic of Aerobic Oxygen", Focus on Nutrition - The Canadian Journal of Health & Nutrition. (Issue No. 21), Burnaby, BC, 1989, Academic Press, N. Y., 1977.

skin, and the hydrochloric acid in our stomachs all react with stabilized oxygen to immediately render the alkalinity harmless to humans."[182]

Contributing Editor Zane Baranowski wrote:

"Stabilized oxygen "...products are made primarily of chlorine, sodium and water, with extra oxygen stabilized in the the water. This is done by replacing chlorine and/ or sodium ions with oxygen molecules. This allows the water to carry larger amounts of oxygen in its whole, stabilized, O2 state. The amount of chlorine in these solutions is small and easily excreted."[183]

James Lembreck, DCH, wrote:

"Stabilized oxygen is often confused with hydrogen peroxide, but has a very different action and is very safe to use."[184]

Almost 30 years ago, while these writers and researchers were using hydrogen peroxide and oxychlorine salts as oxygen supplements, a process control engineer was working diligently on what would become a new generation of stabilized oxygen supplements. This new formula was based on dissolved, yet completely stable, polyatomic oxygen molecules in water rather than oxygen molecules bound to various mineral salts (like the chlorine dioxide molecule). His was a revolutionary concept.

---

[182] McCabe, Ed. Oxygen Therapies: A New Way of Approaching Diseases. Energy Publications, Morrisville, NY (1994).

[183] Baranowski, Zane. "Keep Breathing". Health Freedom News, October 1988: 31-34.

[184] Lembreck, James, D.C.H., C.M.P. "Stabilized Oxygen .. Breathe Easy". Natural Physique, June 1991: 85.

The scientific community defended its position that it was virtually impossible to dissolve and maintain more than about 20 parts per million (ppm) of oxygen in water even under ideal laboratory conditions. Yet, in test after test, the oxygen levels of this new "breed" of stabilized oxygen indicated levels of dissolved oxygen thousands of times more.

This new oxygen stabilizing process was developed by C. B. Smith[185] and his process is still considered "breakthrough" hydro-electrolysis technology where water is broken into its constituent molecular elements of hydrogen (as H_2) and oxygen (O_1). In his process, rather than creating oxygen gas (O_2), which cannot be stabilized and retained in solution, he successfully created polyatomic tetraoxygen (O_4). In this form, the oxygen atoms' electrical bonds are strong enough to keep the atoms together in one single four-oxygen atom molecule. Because of its electrical stability and atomic weight, the O_4 molecules remained in the water at levels that reached 50,000 ppm or more.

Regardless of the fact that some scientists say that this is not possible, they cannot deny that the oxygen-rich solution defies explanation. The original O_4 solution, and its subsequent successor formulations, was also the first stabilized oxygen supplement to possess a nearly balanced pH.[186] This pH measurement is significant because all other competitive stabilized oxygen solutions on the market today, based on the chlorine dioxide (chlorite) molecular oxygen delivery system, have extremely alkaline levels. This makes

---

[185] The original inventor was C.B.Smith. I had the distinct pleasure of knowing and working with him between 1989 and 2004. Mr. Smith was a process control engineer for the National Advisory Committee for Aeronautics (NACA) during the early 1950s, (the precursor agency to NASA,) and he spent nearly 30 years as a Chief Process Control Engineer for Kennecott Utah Copper.

[186] pH values express the acidity or alkalinity of a solution on a scale of 1 to 14. Distilled water is considered the neutral "middle point" solution at a pH of 7.0. The lower the pH value, the more acidic the solution is; the higher the pH value, the more alkaline the solution is.

these other solutions potentially harmful when used in full concentration especially if exposed to the eyes, skin and respiratory system.

Since the introduction of this revolutionary oxygen-rich O_4 solution, a family of even more concentrated stabilized oxygen solutions has appeared. Each succeeding formulation claims it provides even more benefits for specific markets including agricultural, cosmetic, dental, disinfectant and health and nutrition. Yet, in spite of what appears to be the higher levels of dissolved oxygen in these new solutions, these solutions continue to demonstrate low to non-existent toxicity and high efficacy. Most are sold as proprietary, low sodium, trace mineral and essential mineral dietary supplement formulations.

In a limited human-use study on one such solution, conducted by quantum physicist, Dr. James Aker, Ph.D., he concluded:

> *"It is the researcher's opinion that stabilized oxygen results in greater metabolic efficiency which may correlate to significant energy reductions thus prolonging and enhancing the quality of an individual's life. Further, stabilized oxygen, used in conjunction with mineral supplements, may be an excellent therapeutic tool for treating physiological disorders including chronic fatigue syndrome, immune deficiency disorders and several chronic pain related disorders. Regardless of the oxygen delivery system, most of the oxygen supplements on the market today, regardless of the technology, offer varying degrees of physiological benefits. Since the release of the first commercial stabilized oxygen supplement called Halox almost 25 years ago, dozens of other products have been introduced for sale to the health and nutrition industry. Many appear to be variations of the same products and merely marketed under different trade names. Others claim to utilize unique oxygen delivery systems con-*

taining minerals in various forms. The three basic categories of stabilized oxygen solutions are hydrogen peroxide, oxy-halogen formulations (including chlorine dioxide/ chlorite and magnesium peroxide), and mono-atomic dissolved oxygen. All stabilized oxygen dietary supplements fall into one of these three categories."[187]

---

[187] James D. Aker, M.S., P.A., P.P.A., President and C.E.O. of Third State Industries, Inc. Study: "Capillary Martin Microscope Oxygen Saturation Test conducted using Activated Stabilized Oxygen (A02CTM) Solution at 100% Full Concentration", April 10, 1998.

Chapter Eighteen:
Measuring the "Energy Potential" in Oxygenated Water

O.R.P. stands for Oxidation-Reduction Potential. In practical terms, it is a measurement of how much an atom group of atoms, a molecule or an ion, can oxidize another atom, ion or molecule. Sometimes O.R.P. is referred to as the Redox Potential.

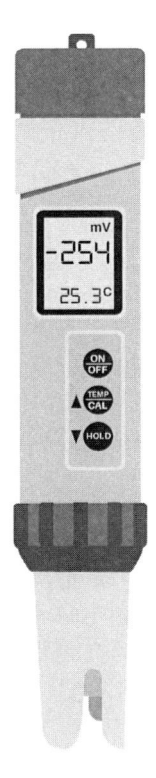

When chemists first used the term in the late 18th Century, the word "oxidation" meant "to combine with oxygen." Back then, it was a "radical" concept. Nearly 200 years ago, people were confused about the nature of matter. It took some brave chemists to prove, for example, that fire did not involve the release of some unknown, mysterious substance, but rather occurred when oxygen combined rapidly with what was being burned.

All matter is composed of molecules. Molecules are made up of tinier particles called atoms. An atom consists of a positively charged nucleus that is surrounded by one or more negatively charged particles called electrons. The positive charges must equal the negative charges so that the atom can maintain electrical neutrality. The majority of an atom's mass[188] is found in its nucleus. This nucleus contains both protons and neutrons. The mass of protons and neutrons are almost equal but they differ in

---

[188] Atomic mass is a characteristic of an atom that is a measure of its size. Mass plays a major role in the chemical properties of elements. Atomic mass is roughly equal to the sum of an atom's individual particles.

their electrical charges. A neutron lacks an electrical charge while a proton has a positive charge. The proton's charge exactly balances the negative charge of a single orbiting electron.

When two atoms are close enough to combine and react chemically to form a chemical bond, it is the electron that determines or "sees" the incoming atom and determines the chemical compatibility. The electrons in the outer most shell of one atom react with the number of electrons in the outer most shell of another atom. Seeking electrical equilibrium, electrons jump from one atom to another, or are shared by both atoms, forming a bond. Therefore, it is the electron that is the key to the chemical behavior of atoms. Neither the neutron nor the proton can rival the significance of this tiny negatively charged particle.

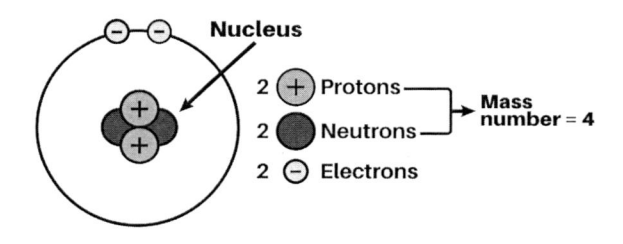

An atoms stability depends on a corresponding balance between electrons (-), protons (+) and neutrons (no charge).

In dealing with human health, a growing field is understanding the nature of "free radicals". As I have described, free radicals are negatively charged atoms or groups of atoms called ions (or anions). The ion is formed by the loss or the gain of one or more electrons. A cation (positive ion), is created by an electron loss. An anion (negative ion), is created by an electron gain. The orbits of the electrons around these ions are called "valences"[189].

The valence of an ion is equal to the number of electrons lost or gained and is indicated by a plus sign (+) for cations and a minus sign (-) for anions. For example, when salt is put into water, it separates into two distinct ions: the cation sodium (Na^+) and the anion chloride (Cl^-). An ionic bond is the chemical link between these two atoms caused by the electrical attractions between their two oppositely-charged ions.

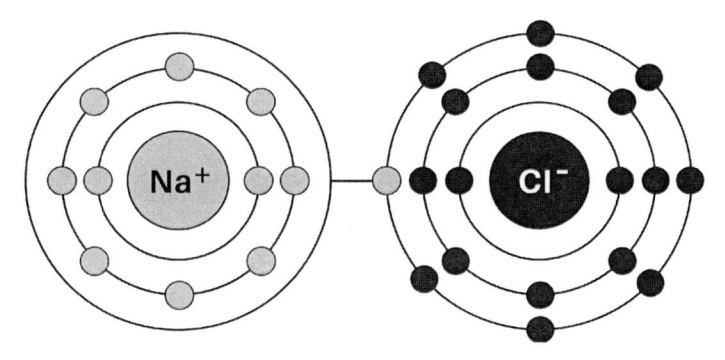

A salt molecule (NaCl), called sodium chloride, separates into two distinct ions when dissolved in water: the sodium cation (Na^+) and the chloride anion (Cl^-)

Oxidation-Reduction is an important concept in understanding chemical reactions involving oxygen. Oxidation is described as the loss of electrons by one atom or molecule and reduction as involving the gain of an electron by another. Both oxidation and reduction occur simultaneously, and in equivalent amounts, during any reaction involving either process.

---

[189] A valence electron is a single electron, or one of two or more electrons, in the outer shell of an atom that is responsible for the chemical properties of that atom.

We can see examples of oxidation all the time in our daily lives. They occur at different speeds. When we see a piece of iron rusting, or a slice of apple turning brown, we are looking at examples of relatively slow oxidation. When we look at a fire, we are witnessing an example of rapid oxidation.

We know that oxidation involves an exchange of electrons between two atoms. The atom that loses an electron in the process is said to be "oxidized." The one that gains an electron is said to be "reduced." In gaining an additional electron, it loses the electrical energy that makes it "hungry" for more electrons.

Oxidation reduction potential in millivolts (mV)	Kill time
450	Infinite
500	1 hour
550	100 seconds
600	10 seconds
650	0 seconds

The amount of contact time needed to oxidize (kill) the pathogenic bacteria Escherichia coli is based on the oxidation reduction potential (O.R.P.) Measurements are in millivolts (mV).

Chemicals like chlorine, bromine, and oxygen, (including singlet oxygen, ozone, diatomic oxygen tetraoxygen, etc.,) are all oxidizers. It is their ability to oxidize - to "steal" electrons from other substances - that makes them great sanitizers. Their atoms and molecules alter the chemical makeup of pathogenic microorganisms and toxic chemicals, and in this process either kill them or decompose them, "burning up" the remains, and leaving less harmless molecules as metabolic by-products. Of course, in the process of oxidizing, all of these oxidizers are reduced - so they lose their ability to further oxidize things.

The polyatomic tetraoxygen molecule (four atoms of oxygen, or O_4,) that was created by C. B. Smith, for example, is extremely unique because the individual singlet oxygen atoms (O_1) are held tightly together in this molecule cluster of four atoms. This four atom oxygen molecule shares an electron at the outer valence of each atom. This sharing of electrons causes each atom to retain the correct charge that holds the four atoms together.

However, each atom is still seeking a remaining electron to balance out its final valence. So when this atom comes into close proximity to organic compounds, or carbon-based microorganisms, it quickly disassociates (splits apart) and steals electrons from the host compound or organism. It is this process of oxidation that either turns the molecule into something less toxic to the body or kills the microorganism.

Potential energy is energy that is stored and ready to be put to work. It's not actually working, but we know that the energy is there if and when we need it. Another word for potential might be pressure. Blow up a balloon, and there is air pressure inside. As long as we keep the end tightly closed, the pressure remains as potential energy. Release the end, and the air inside rushes out, changing from potential (possible) energy to kinetic (in motion) energy.

In electrical terms, potential energy is measured in volts. Actual energy (current flow) is measured in amps. When you put a voltmeter across the leads of a battery, the reading you get is the difference in electrical pressure - the potential - between the two poles. This pressure represents the excess electrons present at one pole of the battery (caused, incidentally, by a chemical reaction within the battery) that is ready to flow to the opposite pole.

When we use the term potential in describing O.R.P., we are actually talking about electrical potential or voltage. We are reading the very tiny voltage generated

O.R.P. in mV	Item Description
-2,000	Hydroxyl Free Radical (OH⁻) -2,000mV
-1,875	
-1,750	Singlet Oxygen (O_1) -1,780 mV
-1,625	
-1,500	Ozone (O_3) -1,520 mV
-1,375	
-1,250	Hydrogen Peroxide / 35% (H_2O_2) -1,300 mV
-1,125	
-1,000	Chlorine (Cl_2) -1,000 mV
-875	Polyatomic Tetraoxygen (O_4) -950 mV Diatomic Oxygen (O_2) -940 mV Hypochlorus Acid (HOCl) -800 mV
-750	Minimum ORP to kill Crystosporidium -800 mV Minimum ORP to kill Yeasts / Molds -750 mV Sodium Hypochlorite ($NaHClO_2$) -690 mV
-625	W.H.O. minimum ORP to disinfecting H_2O -650 mV Sodium Chlorite / 50,000 ppm ($NaClO_2$) -650 mV Minimim ORP to kill Salmonella -650 mV Minimim ORP to kill Poliovirus -650 mV
-500	
-375	Alkalized H_2O -350 mV
-250	Carbon Dioxide (CO_2) -280 mV Cod Liver Oil -200 mV
-125	Fresh Orange Juice -200 mV Green Tea - 180 mV
0	
125	Coffee +175 mV Goji Juice +181 mV Vodka +220 mV
250	Purified Distilled H_2O +320 mV Beer +315 mV Teqiula +315 mV
375	Bottled Water +400 mV Carbonated Soft Drinks +400 mV Tap Water +450 mV
500	

Left-side axis labels: **OXIDATION** (upper) / **REDUCTION** (lower); sub-ranges: Water Sterilization, Pools / Spas, Aquaculture, No Practical Use.

This chart shows the different electrical charges, in millivolts (mV) of different solutions. For any solution to posses antimicrobial properties, it must have an electrical oxidative potential of no less than -650 mV.

when a metal is placed in water in the presence of oxidizing and reducing agents. These voltages give us an indication of the ability of the oxidizers in water to keep it free from organic-based contaminants.

An O.R.P. probe is really a millivolt meter, measuring the voltage across a circuit formed by a reference electrode, constructed of silver wire, (in effect, the negative pole of the circuit), and a measuring electrode constructed of a platinum band (the positive pole), with water in between.

A reference electrode, usually made from silver, is surrounded by salt (electrolyte) solution that produces another tiny voltage. The voltage produced by the reference electrode is constant and stable, so it forms a reference against which the voltage generated by the platinum measuring electrode and the oxidizers in the water may be compared.

The difference in voltage between the two electrodes is what is actually measured by the meter. Modern O.R.P. electrodes are almost always combination electrodes, that is both electrodes are housed in one body - so it appears that it is just one "probe."

Although O.R.P. does not specifically tell you the concentration of an oxidizing agent in parts per million, it does indicate the effectiveness of the agent as an oxidizer. An O.R.P. reading will vary as pH fluctuates. As the pH goes up, the millivolt reading on an O.R.P. meter will go down, indicating that the oxidizing agent is not as effective.

Once the instruments and methods for measuring O.R.P. were developed in the 1960's, researchers began working toward setting standards under which O.R.P. measurements could be used as an accurate gauge to determine water quality. In 1972, the World Health Organization (WHO) adopted an O.R.P. standard for drinking water disinfection at 650 millivolts. That is, the WHO stated that when the oxidation-reduction potential in a body of water measures 650/1,000 (about 2/3) of a volt, the oxidizing agent in the water is active enough to destroy harmful organisms, almost instantaneously.

In Germany, which has the strictest water quality standards in the world, an O.R.P. level of 750 millivolts has been established as the minimum standard for public pools (1982) and spas (1984).

In its 1988 standards for commercial pools and spas, the National Spa & Pool Institute stated that O.R.P. can be used as a "supplemental measurement of proper sanitizer activity" when chlorine or bromine are used as primary disinfectants. The recommended minimum reading under the NSPI standards is 650 millivolts.

During the 1920's, medical scientists and chemists began to discover that the monitoring of electrons (or electron potential) of bodily fluids was just as critical as measuring body pH. In living tissue, oxidation-reduction reactions occur simultaneously or consecutively at the cellular level. The entire purpose for oxidation and reduction is:

- To create high cellular energy in the form of ATP;
- To oxidize or burn up invading pollutants and microorganisms

These two events are so significant that without them our life, as we know it, would cease to exist. ATP energy is, of course, the cellular energy that fuels each and every cell of our bodies. Without the adequate production of ATP, our bodies would rapidly run out of the fuel that enables them to work. When our cells stop functioning, so does our body.

The ability of our cells to oxidize invading pollutants and microorganisms is paramount to survival in a contaminated and polluted world. If the oxidation-reduction reaction were not able to burn up these contaminants and invaders, cellular integrity would most certainly be compromised leading to disease and death.

When blood is loaded with electron energy, because of the presence of oxygen, there is a great potential for life-giving chemical reactions to occur. However, when blood becomes depleted of its electrical oxidizing potential the energy of blood has been spent.

O.R.P. is therefore a measure of energy potential. The more negative the O.R.P., the more electrons are present (in relation to the number of protons), and the more energy that is available. Biological redox reactions are a result of hydrogen being the essential electron donor, and oxygen being the essential electron acceptor.

About Antioxidants

There are tens of thousands of natural compounds that have demonstrated antioxidant activity and just as many natural health products (dietary supplements) on the market with an antioxidant claim.

The basic truth is that the plant and marine kingdom are full of natural compounds with antioxidant activity. These include the flavonoids, a huge category that is further subdivided into more subcategories. Flavonoids include the colorful anthocyanins, (which gives berries their striking colors), quercetin, (which is abundant in apples and onions) and also polymethoxy flavones from citrus fruits. Polymethoxy flavones is another group of antioxidants that have potent anti-cancer activity.

Similarly, various carotenoids, including zeaxanthin from paprika, lutein from marigold flowers and fucoxanthin from algae offer exciting possibilities for health. The antioxidants curcumin, from turmeric root, (which is widely used in Asian cuisine,) and catechins from green tea also exhibit powerful antioxidant effects.

The natural chemical compounds in these plants and organisms are able to quench free radicals generated from oxygen, nitrogen and sulphur, any of which are potentially so reactive they can cause cellular damage as soon as they come into contact with the various compounds in tissues of the body. Especially susceptible to free radical damage is DNA, the lipid molecules of cell membranes, proteins and amino acids that form the structural components of skin, joints and nerve cells.

Scientists have long considered oxidative stress to be a significant contributor to cellular aging and an important factor in being responsible for chronic diseases. It is important to remember that the body is able to defend itself through various mechanisms to counteract oxidative stress.

We do know that the body does not absorb, store or use antioxidants completely. Even more important is calculating how much of an antioxidant is actually absorbed since the body does not absorb 100% of what is being consumed.

in fact, most antioxidants that we 'eat', do not get into the cells at all. We simply absorb the vital nutrients to make energy, and extract only the needed nutrients that we need. That means the oxidative power of free radicals (produced inside the cells) are not affected. We may see quantitative results it in a petri-dish, but it is a completely different matter when we are looking at what happens inside living tissues.

The human organism makes trillions of free radicals every day. The few million molecules of antioxidants that we eat is not anywhere close to the amount we need to counter the number of free radicals being generated. So, if there is such a huge difference in these numbers, why don't we all quickly die from free-radical damage? The reason is that our bodies produce their own antioxidants.

We make Superoxide Dismutase (SOD), Catalase (CAT) and Glutathione (GSH), which are antioxidant enzymes and proteins, that destroy millions of free radicals every second. As we age, our bodies make less of these. Vitamin and mineral supplements assist in filling this gap.

A FINAL WORD FROM THE AUTHOR

Everything is theoretically impossible, until it is done. One could write a history of science in reverse by assembling the solemn pronouncements of highest authority about what could not be done and could never happen.
Robert A. Heinlein

> *The doubters said,*
> *"Man can not fly."*
> *The doers said,*
> *"Maybe, but we'll try."*
> *And finally soared*
> *In the morning glow*
> *While non-believers*
> *Watched from below.*
> *Bruce Lee*

As I stated at the beginning of this book, for almost three decades I have personally witnessed the remarkable results of the power of oxygen in health, wellness and the natural eradication of pathogens that have plagued humankind. Yet, in spite of the overwhelming evidence, the medical and pharmaceutical community, using the F.D.A. as its attack dog, has continued to suppress, frighten and coerce the brave pioneers in this industry.

"Why", anyone with common sense would ask, "is there so much resistance to this modality/therapy?" Even someone not accustomed to entertaining conspiratorial theories has to question the almost rabid-like frenzy coming from the government and the Western medical community.

In my opinion, it has more to do with money than it does with unbelief. The drug industry is huge, not just in income and profits, but also in its influence over the global economy.

"The combined profits for the ten drug companies in the Fortune 500 ($35.9 billion) were more than the profits for all the other 490 businesses put together ($33.7 billion). Over the past two decades the pharmaceutical industry has moved very far from its original high purpose of discovering and producing useful new drugs. Now primarily a marketing machine to sell drugs of dubious benefit, this industry uses its wealth and power to co-opt every institution that might stand in its way, including the US Congress, the FDA, academic medical centers, and the medical profession itself." [190]

Big Pharma is the nickname given to the world's vast and influential pharmaceutical industry and its trade group, the Pharmaceutical Research and Manufacturers of America or PhRMA. These powerful companies make billions of dollars every year by selling drugs and medical devices.

Big Pharma wields enormous influence over the prescription drug and medical device markets around the globe. In the U.S., the industry contributes heavily to the annual budget of the U.S. Food and Drug Administration (FDA), which is charged with regulating drugs and devices made by those same companies.

The industry demonstrates its power, political might and social influence over the nation's governments and agencies, its health care systems, its doctors and hospitals, as well as the psyche of the American people.

The global market for pharmaceuticals topped $1 trillion in sales in 2014. The world's 10 largest drug companies generated $429.4 billion of that revenue. Five of the top 10 companies are headquartered in the U.S.: Johnson & Johnson, Pfizer, Abbot Laboratories, Merck and Eli Lilly.

---

[190] The Truth About the Drug Companies
Marcia Angell, M.D.
http://www.wanttoknow.info/truthaboutdrugcompanies

With the help of staggering profits and 1,100-plus paid lobbyists, the industry has gained powerful leverage on Capitol Hill. From 1998 to 2014, Big Pharma spent nearly $2.9 billion on lobbying expenses — more than any other industry. The industry also doled out more than $15 million in campaign contributions from 2013-14.

But the large amount of cash Big Pharma bestows on government representatives and regulatory bodies is small when compared with the billions it spends each year on direct-to-consumer advertising. The U.S. is one of only two countries in the world whose governments allow prescription drugs to be advertised on TV (the other is New Zealand).

A single manufacturer, Boehringer Ingelheim, spent $464 million advertising its blood thinner Pradaxa in 2011. The following year, the drug passed the $1 billion sales mark. The money spent on this business appears to be well-allocated.[191]

With this much influence, power and money behind them, Big Pharma can easily crush any cost-effective and easily available modality that will cut into their profits. Just consider the fact that last year (2015) over $100 billion dollars was spent by consumers on cancer drugs and it is estimated that expenditures on oncology medicines will grow more than eight percent a year through 2018![192]

If you need further evidence, here's what was published just a few months ago by the Alliance for Natural Health:

---

[191] From: https://www.drugwatch.com/manufacturer/

[192] Cancer drug spending hit $100 billion in 2014. Here's why it'll soon be much higher
Laura Lorenzetti
http://fortune.com/2015/05/08/cancer-drug-spending-100-billion-in-2014-headed-higher/

"Earlier this year we covered a new study conducted at the China Medical University in Taiwan showing how non-drug therapies such as the ketogenic diet[193] and hyperbaric oxygen therapy were being used to cure cancer.

"There is has been a lot of research into the use of hyperbaric oxygen treatment for cancer and other diseases lately. So it should come as no surprise that the FDA, in an obvious effort to protect the lucrative drug market for treating cancer, has issued a statement saying that hyperbaric oxygen therapy is 'not approved' by them for such treatment.

"The agency has just issued a warning to consumers. As is so often the case, what they don't tell you is more important than what they do tell you. The agency's warning begins, 'No, hyperbaric oxygen therapy (HBOT) has been clinically proven to cure or be effective in the treatment of cancer, autism, or diabetes.' But do a quick search on the Internet, and you'll see all kinds of claims for these and other diseases for which the device has not been cleared or approved by FDA.

"HBOT is approved to treat thirteen conditions: decompression sickness, thermal burns, non-healing wounds, necrotizing soft tissue infections (a.k.a. flesh-eating bacterial disease), acute traumatic ischemia (e.g., crush injury, compartment syndrome), radiation tissue damage, smoke inhalation and carbon monoxide poisoning, air or gas embolism, severe blood loss anemia, refractory osteomyelitis, compromised skin grafts, and clostridial myonecrosis (gangrene).

"There are, however, many other conditions that HBOT appears to treat effectively, based on solid or promising research. Licensed physicians and healthcare institutions may legally use an FDA-

---

[193] Study: Ketogenic Diet and Hyperbaric Oxygen Therapy Stops Cancer. http://healthimpactnews.com/2013/study-ketogenic-diet-and-hyperbaric-oxygen-therapy-stops-cancer/

cleared hyperbaric chamber to treat unapproved or 'off-label' diseases and conditions, though it is illegal to promote or advertise such uses."[194]

Ignorance is not "bliss" when it concerns our health and the health of our families. Ignorance may result in more major medical complications and death. Here's what Mike Adams, Editor of one of there largest and most respected natural products web-based newsletters writes:

> "America is a nation of widespread health and nutritional illiteracy. And I'm not just talking about the knowledge gaps of health consumers, either. It's the doctors and health "experts" who have astonishing gaps in knowledge that should be considered basic health information in any first-world nation.
>
> "Parents, too, lack any real literacy in nutrition and health. That's largely because medical journals, health authorities and the mass media actively misinform them about health and nutrition issues, hoping to prevent people from learning how to take care of their own health using simple, natural remedies and cures. So why do conventional medical doctors remain so ignorant of the basics of human health and nutrition? Because medical schools don't teach health. They teach disease, surgery and pharmacology. They offer virtually no material on nutrition, disease prevention or mind-body medicine, so the doctors that graduate from medical school are nutritionally illiterate and lacking basic health knowledge.
>
> "Yet, at the same time, they are being told that they know everything about health and the human body, so they suffer from the most dangerous combination of all: A smug, know-it-all attitude com-

---

[194] FDA Seeks to Restrict Hyperbaric Oxygen Therapy Used in Cancer Treatment. August 26, 2016, Alliance for Natural Health
https://healthimpactnews.com/2013/fda-seeks-to-restrict-hyperbaric-oxygen-therapy-used-in-cancer-treatment/

bined with far-reaching health illiteracy. This is one of the key reasons why America's health care system is such an utter failure -- the people who are supposed to possess more health knowledge than everybody else are the very same people who actually lack it. In a sense, they have been "de-educated" by medical schools and come out knowing less than they did when they entered med school.

"I'm not the only one who thinks this. In fact, you'll find some of these concerns reflected by other doctors who are appalled at the arrogance and health illiteracy of their own peers. For example, a commentary published in the July 14 issue of the Journal of the American Medical Association (JAMA) features Dr. Pronovost, a professor of anesthesiology and critical care medicine at the Johns Hopkins University School of Medicine, explaining how physician arrogance is killing tens of thousands of patients across America today.

"Holistically-trained doctors who went way beyond medical school and taught themselves principles of nutrition often describe their own conventional medical school training as wildly inadequate. Dr Andrew Weil, for example, famously describes his conventional medicine colleagues as 'nutritionally illiterate.'

"And he's right. Most conventional doctors are nutritionally illiterate. So are most parents. And if we wish to change the health future of America, this situation obviously needs to change. Nutrition should be the foundation of med school training, not an afterthought.

"You can't create a healthy nation if the people practicing medicine don't know much about health and nutrition themselves."[195]

---

[195] When it comes to health knowledge, doctors are surprisingly ignorant. Mike Adams. October 11, 2010. NaturalNews.com
http://www.naturalnews.com/030010_doctors_illiteracy.html

Oxygen, so important for all of the metabolic processes in our bodies, is finally being recognized for all of its health benefits and is no longer vilified because of its oxidation potential. The fact that you are reading the last words in this book is another milestone that the individual is taking back the autonomy of his or her body.

The "naysayers" claim that you cannot create a stable, pH balanced and highly concentrated oxygen solution that would be safe to consume. The skeptics said that it was impossible for the human body to extract life-giving oxygen from any solution. You would have to be a "fish with gills". The critics said supplemental oxygen and oxygen-based therapies were marginally beneficial, at best.

Hundreds of thousands of consumers around the world, people just like you and me, have demonstrated that these so-called experts have been, and continue to be, wrong. Even so, they will not retract their rhetoric or admit that all they are espousing is merely biased opinions that have no real basis in personal studies, research or clinical testing.

My simple goal in writing this book was to expose the bias and to provide support to those with more open minds who just ask for honest answers and new alternatives so their lives can be more productive and enjoyable.

Thank you for sharing this time with me. You've opened yourself up to new concepts, more possibilities as well as, I hope, a healthier and longer life.

And, if you would like to share your thoughts and experiences with me, I would be honored to read them. Just drop me a note at <droxygen@oxigenesis.com>.

Stephen R. Krauss, Ph.D.
2017

Appendix One:
Oxygen and Nutritional Glossary

A

Acid-Alkaline Balance: The body's pH, a measurement of the body's acidity or alkalinity, is 80% alkaline and 20% acidic by design. Most diets, even those of vegetarians, are 75% acidic and 25% alkaline. Excesses in either area result in a lack of hydrochloric acid (HCl) in the stomach which reduces the production of pancreatic enzymes that are important in the digestion process. Undigested or partially digested food sits in the stomach and the intestines and ferments (rots). This putrid mass travels through almost 40 feet of intestines spreading its toxic poisons. This results in the poor assimilation of nutrients from consumed foods and an increase of toxins in the blood stream. Coffee, tea, soft drinks and other foods radically alter the body's pH to an acidic value. A highly acidic body will provide an environment where yeasts, viruses, parasites and cancer cells can thrive. In addition, bodies that suffer acidic states for prolonged periods of time consume the body's stored reserves of sodium, calcium, potassium and magnesium. This reserve of minerals is crucial as they act as catalysts that activate the enzymes that digest and assimilate food.

Acid/Base: Acids are ionic compounds (a compound with a positive or negative charge) that break apart in water to form a hydrogen ion (H^+). The strength of an acid is based on the concentration of H^+ ions in the solution. The more H^+ the stronger the acid. Bases are ionic compounds that break apart to form a negatively charged hydroxide ion (OH^-) in water. The strength of a base is determined by the concentration of Hydroxide ions (OH^-). The greater the concentration of OH^- ions the stronger the base. When acids and bases are added to each other they react to neutralize each other if an equal number of hydrogen and hydroxide ions are present.

Actin: A muscle protein localized in the I band of the myofibrils. It is responsible, along with myosin, for the contraction and relaxation of muscles.

ADP: Adenosine diphosphate ($C_{10}H_{15}N_5O_{10}P_2$) is a nucleotide that is present in, and vital to the energy processes of all living cells. During biological oxidations energy is stored in the ATP molecule as ADP. ADP is converted to back into ATP, which later converts back to ADP, releasing the energy needed for muscular contractions and biosynthesis.

Aerobic: A condition or state that contains oxygen. Aerobic organisms are ones that can only survive (live) and only reproduce in an oxygen-rich environment or atmosphere. The opposite state or condition is called "anaerobic".

Allotrope: Each of two or more different physical forms in which an element can exist. Graphite, charcoal, and diamond are all allotropes of carbon.

Alveolar Sac: Alveolar sacs contain tiny pouches called alveoli, whose primary function is gas diffusion. These clusters of alveoli have thin walls that allow oxygen to pass easily from the lungs into the bloodstream and carbon dioxide to flow from the blood to the lungs so it can exit the body. These alveoli are the smallest types of lung tissue, and one of the most important. In addition to being the primary means by which oxygen enters and carbon dioxide escapes the bloodstream, these small pouches of air are also the reason why the lungs do not totally collapse when a person breathes out. This is because they contain a cell that secretes a special chemical to lower the surface temperature to prevent lung collapse. The alveoli also contain other cells that secrete chemicals to attack and remove any foreign objects in the lungs, such as dust, dirt and other debris.

Amino Acid: The basic building block used by every cell in the body to manufacture proteins. What distinguishes one protein from another is the way the cells assemble amino acids into proteins. There are over 20 different amino acids that combine in different ways and combinations to make all of the proteins we need. These proteins are divided into two groups: essential amino acids, (there are eight of these that cannot be manufactured by the body and must be derived from the foods we eat,) and non-essential amino acids, (there are twelve of these and they are manufactured by the body.)

Anabolism: The chemical process in the body where a more complex substance is built from simpler ones. This process requires energy which cannot happen without the presence of oxygen. An example of an anabolic process is the synthesis of proteins from amino acids.

Anaerobic: A condition or state that lacks oxygen. Almost all pathogenic (harmful) organisms that cause disease are anaerobic. These include bacteria, viruses, yeasts, molds, fungi and parasites. When these organisms are placed in an oxygen-rich state, these organisms die.

Anaerobic glycolysis: Anaerobic glycolysis is the conversion of glucose to lactate that occurs when limited amounts of oxygen (O_2) are available. Anaerobic glycolysis is only an effective means of energy production during short, intense exercise, and provides energy for a very brief period ranging from 10 seconds to 2 minutes.

Anode: The anode is the positively charged electrode. The anode attracts electrons or anions. The anode may be a source of positive charge or an electron acceptor.

Anion: A negatively charged ion (See "ion.")

Antibiotics: An anti-bacterial substance used against an organisms created from or out of another living organism. Penicillin is a relatively non-toxic acidic substance extracted from the green mold Penicillin notatum that has very powerful anti-bacterial properties.

Antioxidant: A group of vitamins, minerals and enzymes that the body uses to protect itself against the formation of free radicals. (See "free radicals".) Antioxidant molecules include vitamins A, C, E, the B-family, gamma-linoleic acid (GLA) and L-cysteine.

Artery: One of the main tubular-shaped branching vessels from the heart that carries the oxygen and nutrient-rich blood to the organs and cells in the body.

Arthritis: An inflammation of a joint in the body associated with pain, swelling, stiffness and redness. It is believed that arthritis is caused by bacterial infections. Oxygen therapies are the newest approach to relieving both the symptoms and the cause of most types of arthritis.

Atom: A unit of matter, the smallest unit of an element, having all the characteristics of that element and consisting of a dense, central, positively charged nucleus surrounded by a system of electrons. The entire structure has an approximate diameter of 10^{-8} centimeter and characteristically remains undivided in chemical reactions except for limited removal, transfer, or exchange of certain electrons.

A.T.P. (Adenosine TriPhosphate: ($C_{10}H_{16}N_5O_{13}P_3$): This chemical compound, is a small molecule comprised of carbon, hydrogen, nitrogen, oxygen and phosphorus. It is the essential by-product of the combining oxygen and glucose in the cells in our bodies. ATP is the "energy pack" used for cellular metabolism. Without A.T.P. the cells cannot create heat nor can they function properly.

B

Bacteria: A large group of primarily one-celled microorganisms from the class Schizomycetes that are usually parasitic or saprophytic (living on dead or decaying matter). Bacteria are spherical in shape (coccus), rod-shaped (bacillus) or spiral or thread-like shaped (spirillum). Many bacteria cause diseases like food poisoning and pneumonia, while others are very active in food fermentation and the conversion of dead organic matter into nutrients for plants.

Basophils: Basophils are white blood cells that function as the signal core to let the immune system know that heparin needs to be released into the blood stream. Heparin is the substance that prevents the blood from coagulating. Heparin also functions as a substance that removes fat (cholesterol) particles from the blood stream.

Benign and Malignant Tumors: There are two main classifications of tumors: benign and malignant. A benign tumor is a tumor that does not invade its surrounding tissue or spread throughout the body. A malignant tumor is a tumor that invades its surrounding tissue and spreads throughout the body.

Bilirubin: Bilirubin is the waste product of the decomposition and breakdown of red blood cells and hemoglobin. Bilirubin is transported by the body to the liver where it is converted to bile.

Bioavailable Oxygen (Dissolved Oxygen): The extent to which oxygen is taken up by a specific tissue or organ after administration; the proportion of the dose of oxygen that reaches the systemic circulation intact after administration by a route other than intravenous. Also called systemic availability.

Blood: In mammals, blood is usually a deep red, sticky fluid that circulates through the thousands of miles of veins, arteries and capillaries in the body. Blood is manufactured in the marrow of bones. Blood's main function is to serve as the body's transportation system for nutrients, oxygen and wastes from cellular metabolism. It is called the "river of life" because within this ever-flowing river is everything the body needs to sustain itself and also fight off disease. Almost 95% of the blood is actually a somewhat clear, slightly saline (salty) liquid called the "plasma". The blood also contains three types of blood cells: the red blood cells (erythrocytes), white blood cells (leukocytes) and platelets (thrombocytes). Each of these blood cells has a specific and important function to maintain life.

Blood Plasma: Plasma is the clear, straw-colored liquid portion of blood that remains after red blood cells, white blood cells, platelets and other cellular components are removed. It is the single largest component of human blood, comprising about 55 percent, and contains water, salts, enzymes, antibodies and other proteins.

Blood Vessels: (See "Veins, Arteries and Capillaries".)

C

Cancer: A disease whereby normal, healthy cells alter their metabolic functioning from aerobic (respiration) to anaerobic (fermentation). Researchers now believe that cancer develops when the body has been deprived for long periods of an adequate supply of oxygen (hypoxemia). The scientific evidence strongly suggests that, unlike normal cells in the body, cancer cells thrive in a low-body oxygen state. As far back as 1956, Nobel prize winner Dr. Otto Warburg found that chemicals accumulating in the tissues of the body cause 80% of all cancers.

Candida: Candida (short for Candida albicans) is a small, oval-shaped budding fungus that causes infections in both men and women. Candida infects the digestive tract and can spread throughout the entire body resulting in systemic infection. Candida is usually controlled by the friendly, aerobic bacteria Acidophilus that consumes Candida as a Primary food source. If allowed to grow out of control, Candida can produce significant amounts of toxins as part of its metabolic wastes. These toxins cause fatigue, dizziness, constipation, diarrhea and cramping. Candida infections can also cause liver damage as well as damage to the nervous system. Candida can impair the immune and circulatory systems and suppress hormone production in women. Most physicians continue to treat Candida (vaginal yeast) infections in women with medications (drugs) that suppress the symptoms but do not stop the cause. Candida thrives on carbohydrates, sugar yeasts and fermented foods in a low oxygen environment in the body. Many individuals who suffer the symptoms of Candida infections do not realize they are infected with this yeast and are feeding it every day with the foods they eat. Stabilized oxygen and other oxygen therapies have proved to be a very natural and successful alternative therapy to traditional drugs in controlling and eliminating Candida infections.

Capillaries: The smallest blood vessels that deliver oxygen to the cells. If capillaries become clogged or damages, vital nutrients cannot be delivered to the cells resulting in diminished cellular health. Cells starved of oxygen for prolonged periods of time either die or, as described by Nobel Prize winner Dr. Otto Warburg, their metabolism changes and the cells become cancerous.

Capsid: Capsid is the protein shell of a virus particle surrounding its nucleic acid.

Carbohydrates: A group of substances that provide the body with one of its two main sources of energy. (The other group is fats). There are three main types of carbohydrates: monosaccharides (which include sucrose, galactose and fructose,) disaccharides (which include sucrose, lactose and maltose,) and polysaccharides (which include starch and cellulose). Oxygen combines with glucose, the simplest form of sugar derived from carbohydrates to create the energy needed for all cellular metabolic functions. The body will break down all complex carbohydrates into glucose and glycogen (Glycogen is stored as an energy reserve fuel in fat cells.)

Carbon Dioxide: Carbon dioxide (CO_2) is the main waste product of cellular metabolism. It is created when glucose is combined with oxygen to make energy for the cell. After the red blood cells release their life-giving oxygen to the cells, the hemoglobin receptors pick up CO_2 to return these molecules to the lungs where they can be expelled.

Carcinogen: Carcinogens are substances that prevent the body from producing metabolic energy and which facilitate the rise of cancerous cell growth. These can include pollutants (such as tobacco tars, unsaturated oils, carbon monoxide, chemical additives to foods, etc.), electrical factors, which include excessive exposure to X-rays, microwaves, fluorescent lights, radio waves and ultra-violet light. Electrical signals can destroy critical chemical bonds within the cells. Psychological factors include prolonged stress which drains the body of nutrients and energy and weakens the immune system.

Catabolism: The process whereby the body breaks down complex substances into simpler components that the body can use for normal metabolism. Glycogen, a more complex sugar (carbohydrate), is catabolized into glucose, the simplest sugar, which is combined with oxygen in the cells to produce energy.

Cathode: The cathode is the negatively charged electrode. The cathode attracts cations or positive charge. The cathode is the source of electrons or an electron donor. It may accept positive charge. Because the cathode may generate electrons, which typically are the electrical species doing the actual movement, it may be said that cathodes generate charge or that current moves from the cathode to the anode. This can be confusing, because the direction of current would be defined by the way a positive charge would move. The movement of charged particles is called the "current".

Cation: A positively charged (+) ion. Cations get their names from the fact that during the electrolysis process, these ions travel in the solution to the positively charged cathode. (See "ion".)

Cell: The basic and most simplest living unit of our bodies. Every organ is an aggregate of millions of living cells held together by a supporting foundation called "intercellular supporting structures." Every cell, regardless of where it is in the body, has a specific function. All cells must have a sufficient supply of oxygen to combine with carbohydrates, fats and/or proteins to release energy for cellular functions. It is estimated that we have 25 trillion red blood cells and 75 trillion other cells in our bodies. Whenever a cell is damaged or destroyed, the surrounding cells usually generate new cells until the appropriate number of cells are present.

Chemotherapy: A traditional medical procedure whereby extremely toxic drugs are used to kill cancer cells. Unfortunately, these drugs are not selective and have significant side effects on normal tissues. Chemotherapy drugs reduce or destroy the cell's ability to reproduce itself. These drugs affect the bone marrow and halt the production of both red and white blood cells. Chemotherapy drugs also affect the intestinal lining, the hair follicles, the mouth and other organs.

Chloride: A compound in which chlorine has combined with another substance, usually minerals like sodium, magnesium, potassium, etc. Chloride, as a negatively charged ion (Cl^-), is a very important part of the body's metabolic cycle and is recognized by the F.D.A. as an essential nutrient for the body.

Chlorine: Both the proper chemical name, as well as the description of a class, of a highly toxic and carcinogenic gas that easily dissolves in water. While the beneficial side of chlorine is that it kills (oxidizes) pathogenic microbes, it also reacts with humic acid in the body to form trihalomethane (like chloroform) which is suspected of causing numerous degenerative diseases. Chlorine, when it has lost an electron and is bound to certain minerals, forms a chloride ion. Chloride is an essential part of the body's metabolic cycle.

Chlorine Dioxide (Chlorite): Chlorine dioxide (ClO_2), also called "chlorite", is created when chlorine atoms combine with oxygen to form a relatively stable oxy-halogen molecule. Chlorite is a very strong oxidizing agent and is used in the paper and tanning industry as a bleaching agent. Chlorine dioxide is also used to purify (disinfect) waste water as a substitute for chlorine. In the last 20 years it has become popular as a stabilized oxygen dietary supplement competing with hydrogen peroxide. Caution should be used when consuming chlorite as it is typically quite alkaline and can burn the skin, eyes, and delicate membranes in the mouth, esophagus, and respiratory tract. Most chlorine dioxide supplements require the product to be diluted before consumption.

Circulatory System: This is the blood's "highway" in the body. The circulatory system is broken down into two systems which describe the direction of the blood flow. The systemic circulatory system is the system that supplies oxygen-rich blood to the entire body, except the lungs, and then returns the blood back to the lungs to release carbon dioxide. The circulatory system includes the aorta (the body's main artery), arterioles (smaller arteries), capillaries, veins and venules (smaller veins). Veins are very different than arteries because they have one-way valves that prevent the blood from flowing backward and are arranged in the body so that the blood flow can only be in one direction towards the heart. The circulatory system also takes a detour to the liver (called the portals circulatory system). This is where capillaries carrying nutrient-rich blood from the stomach, intestines and other digestive organs all meet together in one place. The liver then processes these nutrients, stores them, or allows them to pass back into the systemic circulatory system. The second part of the circulatory system is the pulmonary circulatory system which is solely responsible for re-oxygenating the blood and serves as the source of oxygen and nutrients for the lungs.

Coenzyme Q10: This enzyme, manufactured in our bodies, works with other enzymes to support the body's bio-energetic functions. Coenzyme Q10 appears to be a mild immune system stimulant and research indicates that this enzyme affects the heart's pumping action as well as its electrical functioning. It is also believed that coenzyme Q10 lowers blood pressure.

Cofactor: A cofactor is a non-protein chemical compound. It is bound to the protein and it is needed in the biological activity of the protein. Another term for them are 'helper molecules' because they help in biochemical transformations. There are two types of cofactors: Coenzymes and Prosthetic groups. Coenzymes are cofactors that are bound loosely to an enzyme. Prosthetic groups are cofactors that are bound tightly to an enzyme.

Colostrum: Colostrum is considered to be Nature's perfect food. It is the "pre-milk" or "first milk" substance produced in the breasts by all mammals during the first 24 hours of lactation. Colostrum provides a newborn infant with immune and growth hormone factors and is the perfect combination of vitamins, minerals, amino acids and proteins to insure the health, vitality and growth of a newborn. Colostrum contains hydrogen peroxide which easily breaks down into water and oxygen. Many researchers believe that this additional oxygen helps infant immune systems fight off pathogens. Bovine (cow) colostrum contains higher levels of all vital nutrients than human colostrum and is harvested under strict F.D.A. and U.S.D.A. guidelines for use as a human dietary supplement. When taken orally or topically, colostrum is very beneficial in strengthening the immune system of in fighting off illness.

Connective Tissues: The body is a structure that composed of different parts including the skeleton, muscles, internal organs and the skin. These components are bound together in a tight package with all parts joined together by connective tissues. Connective tissue is two components: cells and a matrix. The types of cells vary depending on the type of tissue they support. The matrix is the substance in which the cells are embedded and may be fluid, semifluid, gelatinous or protein fibers (collagen fibers are very strong and provide flexibility, elastic fibers are very stretchy and assume their original shape after being stretched, and reticular fibers are very thin and provide support for many soft organs and blood vessels.)

Cytochrome: Any of a class of usually colored proteins that play important roles in oxidative processes and energy transfer during cell metabolism and cellular respiration. Cytochromes are electron carriers. They contain a heme (iron-based) group and are similar in structure to hemoglobin and chlorophyll.

Cytoplasm and Protoplasm: The jellylike material that makes up much of a cell inside the cell membrane, and, in eukaryotic cells, surrounds the nucleus. The organelles of eukaryotic cells, such as mitochondria, the endoplasmic reticulum, and (in green plants) chloroplasts, are contained in the cytoplasm. The cytoplasm and the nucleus make up the cell's protoplasm. Cytoplasm and protoplasm are two terms that describe the living part of the cells. To be specific, Cytoplasm is the cell substance between the cell membrane and the nucleus, which contains the cytosol, organelles, cytoskeleton, and various particles while protoplasm is the living content of a cell that is surrounded by the cell membrane. The protoplasm is composed of the nucleus, cell membrane, and the cytoplasm. Therefore, cytoplasm is a part of the protoplasm. This is why the names of these two components are often used interchangeably. However, as explained above, there exists a distinct difference between cytoplasm and protoplasm. The main difference between cytoplasm and protoplasm can be described as the presence of the nucleus; protoplasm consists of the nucleus while cytoplasm does not.

D

Dietary Supplements vs. O.T.C. (Over the Counter Drugs): Dietary supplements are foodstuffs, which differ from foodstuffs for regular use by the high content of vitamins, minerals or other substances with nutritional or physiological effects and which have been manufactured in order to supplement regular diet of the consumer to achieve a level beneficial for his/her health. This implies that they are not indented for the treatment or prevention of diseases. Unlike dietary supplements, O.T.C. medicinal products are, prior to their placement on the market, subjected to authorization procedures within the scope of which the product quality, safety and efficacy for the defined therapeutic or preventive indications are evaluated. As for the evaluation of efficacy of a medicinal product, it is required that the efficacy must be evidenced by relevant clinical studies the conduct of which has to comply with the tight criteria established by legal regulations.

Diffusion: Diffusion is the action of molecules moving from an area of high concentration to an area of lower concentration.

Digestive System: The digestive system is designed to break food down into its basic chemical components, (vitamins, minerals, amino acids, proteins, sugars, etc.) These component molecules are then absorbed into the blood stream and used for the metabolic processes of the cells and organs. The digestive tract consists of the mouth, pharynx, esophagus, stomach, intestines, duodenum, jejunum, ileum, cecum, colon, rectum and anus. The associated digestive organs include the salivary glands, liver and pancreas.

Dissolved Oxygen: Dissolved oxygen (DO) refers to microscopic bubbles of gaseous oxygen (O_2) that are mixed in water and available to aquatic organisms for respiration, a critical process for almost all organisms. Primary sources of

DO include the atmosphere and aquatic plants.

Disease: A condition where the body's health is in jeopardy. Disease is caused primarily because of a lack of cellular oxygen, the inability of the cell to use oxygen, a lack or an excess of nutrients, or the body's inability to control or eliminate wastes or toxic substances.

DO_2: See "Oxygen Delivery".

D.S.H.E.A.: The Dietary and Supplement Health Education Act (D.S.H.E.A.) was passed by congress in 1996 and went into law on January 1, 1997. The F.D.A. attempted to control and regulate dietary supplements under pressure from the medical and pharmaceutical industries. In response to the F.D.A.'s proposals, consumers all over the country reacted and forced legislators to protect their rights to choose alternative nutritional approaches without restrictions from the government. This law defines the classification of dietary supplements as well as government's limited role in regulating these nutritional items.

E

Electrolyte: A substance that disassociates (breaks down) into ions when fused or when dissolved in a solution and thus will conduct electricity. Within the body, electrolytes play an essential role in the structure and working of every cell as well as maintaining fluid and acid-base balance. The most important electrolytes are: (1) sodium, a key water-balance regulator and necessary for the normal functioning of both muscles and nerves; (2) potassium, associated with acid-base balance and the main constituent of cytoplasm in the cells; (3) calcium, important for blood clotting and for normal muscle physiology; (4) magnesium and chloride, essential for the chemical changes required for all body functions.

Electron (Negatron): An extremely small part of each atom associated with the atom's electrical field or charge. It can be either free (not attached to any atom), or bound to the nucleus of an atom. An abundance of electrons surrounding an atom leads to a negative charge and a lack of electrons results in a positive charge. Electrons circle the nucleus of an atom in orbits representing energy levels. The larger the spherical shell or orbit, the higher the energy contained in the electron.

Emphysema: A chronic obstructive pulmonary disease (COPD) that affects the lung tissue and prevents oxygen from being transferred into the blood stream. Since 1982, diseases of the lungs in the U.S. alone has increased more than 40%. It is now the fourth leading cause of death in the U.S. killing over 85,000 people each year. The main reason for this increase is the rise of cigarette smoking among Americans after World War II. Research clearly shows that smoking causes emphysema in over 80% of all individuals who do smoke. The chemicals, gasses and tars in tobacco smoke block the production of a necessary protein called alphal-antitrypsin (AAT). Loss of AAT's protection allows other enzymes to destroy the elastic fibers in the air sacs in the lungs. Now, fifty years after the end of the war, smoking's progressive lung destruction is taking its toll. Other causes of emphysema include prolonged exposure to industrial fumes, (especially those from coal mines and rock quarries,) and exposure to high levels of smog.

Endocrine System: The endocrine system is a collection of glands which produce hormones. Hormones regulate metabolism, growth and sexual development. The main glands that make up this system are: (1) the pituitary gland, which stimulates the adrenals, thyroid and gonads as well as affects skin pigmentation and growth hormones; (2) the thyroid gland, which stimulates metabolism, body heat production and bone growth; (3) the parathyroid gland, which regulates the levels of calcium in the blood; (4) the adrenal glands, which when stimulated by the pituitary glands maintain the blood pressure and the salt balance of the body; (5) the pancreas, which secretes insulin and glucagon which controls the use of glycogen for cell energy production; (6) the ovaries, which produce estrogen and progesterone and thus influence female physiology; (7) the testes which produce testosterone that stimulates sperm production and the development of male physiology.

Endurance: Endurance is the ability to repeat a series of muscle contractions without fatiguing. Muscle endurance is different from cardiovascular endurance because it involves the muscle fatiguing rather than a limitation in the amount of oxygen being supplied or utilized by the muscles. Muscular endurance is one of the main fitness components, important for success in many sports. Muscle endurance plays a very important role in sports such as rowing. In many other sports, including field team sports, good muscle endurance is also an important part of the overall fitness profile.

Enzyme: Stamina, energy levels and the strength of the immune system are directly related to the level of enzymes in the body. An enzyme is a protein that acts as a catalyst by increasing the rate at which chemical reactions occur. The human body contains over 10,000 different enzymes. At the body's normal temperature, very few biochemical reactions proceed at a significant rate without the presence of an enzyme. Like all catalysts, an enzyme does not control the direction of the reaction but rather increases the rates of the forward and reverse reactions proportionally. As we get older, the levels of enzymes decrease and disease gains a stronger foothold. Enzymes are complex organic compounds that accelerate (catalyze) the transformation of other substances in the body into substances that the body can use for metabolism. There are three types of enzymes: (1) digestive enzymes, which are secreted by the pancreas, stomach and small intestines; (2) food enzymes, which we obtain from raw, uncooked fruits, vegetables, sprouts, soaked seeds and nuts. Cooking destroys these enzymes; (3) metabolic enzymes, which regulate the functions of the blood, tissues and organs. Vitamins and minerals cannot be used by the body unless the proper enzymes are present.

E.P.A.: Environmental Protection Agency. A U.S. regulatory agency originally established to monitor water and air quality to protect citizens from pollution.

Eosinophils: Eosinophils are white blood cells that play an important role in reducing contamination in the blood stream that cause allergic reactions. They are also present in increased numbers whenever the body is suffering from parasitic infestation.

Essential Mineral: It is foolish to believe that the foods we consume today supply all of the nutrients essential to optimum health. Foods of all kinds are the end product of over-processed manufacturing and preparation and have been stripped of vital nutrients, especially vitamins and minerals, which are essential for normal body functions. The federal government has established the recommended daily allowance (RDA) for minerals to maintain normal health. These essential minerals include selenium, magnesium, calcium, zinc, iron, sodium and potassium.

Extracellular Fluid: This is the fluid in the spaces outside or surrounding the cells. Cells are considered to be in a "dry state" when there is only enough extracellular fluid to fill the small spaces and crevices between each cell. Edema is the condition where there is too much fluid between the cells. This excess fluid can choke the cells and cause pressure damage to the blood vessels and nerves.

F

Facultative Anaerobe: A microorganism that can live and grow with or without molecular oxygen.

Fascia: Fascia is the system of connective tissue fibers that lay just under the surface of our skin. Under a microscope, fascia is highly organized in a mesh formulation of tubules filled with water, and its job is to attach, stabilize, enclose and separate muscles and internal organs. Fascia is wrapped throughout the body on "lines of pull." It connects toes to brow in one uninterrupted sheet of fascia, and fingers to chest and neck. The heart fascia is connected at the collarbone, which connects to the arm and fingers. It coils around the bones, muscle fibers, muscle bundles, organs, arteries, veins and nerves, applying tension and compression to the body material it surrounds.

Fats: Fats provide the body with the most concentrated form of fuel energy. Fats consist of fatty acids which contain carbon, hydrogen and very few oxygen atoms. Fats fall into two main groups: saturated and unsaturated. Saturated fatty acids contain the highest concentration of hydrogen atoms and are the basic components of meat and dairy products. Unsaturated fats are those that do not contain a complete or full bonding of hydrogen atoms at each of the available receptor sites on the molecules. Vegetable fats (oils) are unsaturated fats.

F.D.A.: The U.S. Food and Drug Administration. The F.D.A. is a U.S. federal regulatory agency that controls the pharmaceutical, food production, food processing, food supplement and drug industries in the U.S. The F.D.A.'s powers are sweeping and control every area of the health care profession, including hospitals, physicians, medical equipment, therapies, nutritional, over-the-counter drugs, etc.

Free Radical: Free radicals are unstable atoms or groups of atoms (molecules) that can cause damage to our cells, impair our immune system and can eventually lead to infections and various degenerative diseases. Free radicals have both beneficial functions in attacking pathogenic microbes in the body as well as a cumulative detrimental affect. There are three well-documented groups of free radicals: the superoxide, the hydroxyl and the peroxide. Any of these may be formed by exposure to radiation, toxic chemicals, over-exposure to ultraviolet light, or as a result of our normal metabolic processes including the conversion of fat molecules into simpler sugars for fuel for energy. Free radicals are kept in check naturally in the body by free radical scavengers (called antioxidants) which neutralize the free radicals as they are produced. Four key enzymes function in this way. They are superoxide dismutase (SOD), methione reductase, catalase and glutathione peroxidase. All are produced as needed by a healthy body. In addition, other antioxidants include the vitamins A, E, C, the B family and the mineral selenium.

Fungus (Fungi): In human physiology, fungi are a group of living plants, unicellular or multi-cellular in form, that are devoid of chlorophyll and reproduce by means of releasing spores. Fungi live off of dead or decaying matter. In some cases, where the surface (skin) cells have become diseased, damaged or health has been impaired, pathogenic fungi can find a host medium and thus thrive.

G

Glucose: A simple sugar ($C_6H_{12}O_6$) which is absolutely critical in the production of energy in every living cell in the body. Glucose is combined with oxygen in the cell to produce A.T.P. (see "A.T.P.") which is the energy source for cellular metabolism.

Glycogen: A more complex sugar (starch) than glucose that is usually stored in either the liver or in fat cells. Glycogen is the energy reserve fuel for the body. As glucose is depleted, the body draws on this reserve and breaks down the glycogen molecule into glucose which the cells can then use to produce energy.

Glycolysis: Glycolysis literally means "splitting sugars." In glycolysis, glucose (a six carbon sugar) is split into two molecules of a three-carbon sugar. Glycolysis yields two molecules of ATP (free energy containing molecule), two molecules of pyruvic acid and two "high energy" electron carrying molecules of NADH. Glycolysis can occur with or without oxygen. In the presence of oxygen, glycolysis is the first stage of cellular respiration. Without oxygen, glycolysis allows cells to make small amounts of ATP. This process is called fermentation. While glycolysis takes place in the cytosol of the cell's cytoplasm, the next step of cellular respiration called the citric acid cycle, occurs in the matrix of cell mitochondria.

Granulocyte: A family of white blood cells that include neutrophils, basophils and eosinophils. Also called "polymorphonuclear leukocytes". They are called granulocytes because the cells look like they are filled with small granules when viewed under a microscope.

Ground State: An atom is in a ground state when all of the electrons in an atom are at their lowest energy levels. In an excited state, electrons spread out to higher energy levels, and not all are in their lowest levels. A ground state atom possesses electrons in its lowest energy orbitals. This state has the lowest potential energy and is more stable than an atom in an excited state. An example of an atom that has electrons in its ground state is hydrogen. Hydrogen has two electrons filling its first potential energy level. In an excited state, electrons do not fill their lowest energy orbitals. Molecules and atoms can obtain outside energy, resulting in a shift of an electron to a highest energy orbital. Excited state electrons are less stable than those in ground state and have more than minimum potential energy. When atoms are not in their ground state, they may revert to it, giving off energy as they return to the lower energy state.

H

Hemoglobin: Hemoglobin is the respiratory pigment in each red blood cell. Hemoglobin's main component is iron and hemoglobin's main function is to react with oxygen from the lungs to form oxyhemoglobin. This new molecule is then transported through the blood stream to the capillaries where it is released for the cells to use for respiration and metabolism. Once hemoglobin releases its oxygen molecule, it picks up carbon dioxide and transports this waste gas back to the lungs where it is replaced with another oxygen molecule.

Holistic: In 1926, the South African philosopher, Jan Christian Smuts originated the concept "holistic" to mean "whole". Many today refer to holistic as "wholistic" and use the terms interchangeably to mean "whole", "holy" and "healthy". At the basis of holistic medicine is the fact that each of us is responsible for our own health and that preventing disease and sickness is far better than fighting off illness. The goal is "wellness" not just the absence of disease. Physicians and health practitioners are "partners" in maintaining a healthy body, mind and spirit.

Homeopathy: The term "homeopathy" comes from the Greek words "homeosis", meaning similar, and "pathos", meaning suffering or sickness. Homeopathy is thus an alternative approach to health based on the law of similars, or as Hippocrates wrote, "like cures like". Homeopathic remedies contain small doses of natural substances that come from plants, animals and/ or minerals that normally would cause illness or a physiological reaction if taken in larger amounts. The alternative approach works by stimulating the body's own natural defenses and allowing the body to heal itself and helping the body to maintain a natural balance. In traditional medicine, an allergy or flu shot is a homeopathic remedy for preventing disease.

Hormones: A group of chemicals, produced by the organs, (a gland or tissue,) and released into the blood stream that has a specific and unique effect on tissues or organs somewhere else in the body. Hormones control a variety of body functions including growth, response to illness, stress and disease, as well as sexual development. The more important hormone producing glands and tissues include the adrenal glands, gonads, pancreas, thyroid, parathyroid, pituitary and placenta. The kidneys, brain and intestines also secrete hormones.

Hydrogen Peroxide: Hydrogen peroxide (H_2O_2) is merely a water molecule that has an added oxygen atom attached to it ($H_2O + O_1 > H_2O_2$). Hydrogen peroxide is reported to have excellent oxygenating and oxidizing qualities for use in a variety of applications including disinfecting, cosmetics and oxygen therapies. Hydrogen peroxide is also naturally produced by the body as an instrumental part of the immune system's defense mechanisms against invading pathogens. Hydrogen peroxide is also a key ingredient in colostrum, the first milk consumed by infants.

Hydrolysis: A chemical decomposition in which a compound is split into other compounds by reacting with water.

Hypoxemia: The condition where there is a less than adequate supply of oxygen for the cells and tissues of the body which predisposes an individual to a number of degenerative diseases including circulatory problems, digestive disorders and even cancer. When insufficient oxygen is available in the body and blood stream, carbon monoxide (CO) is formed and is not easily eliminated. CO forms a very strong bond with hemoglobin and is not easily displaced by O_2. Thus the level of available oxygen declines preventing the cells from producing the energy necessary for healthy metabolism. Toxins begin to build up, organs get irritated, the body temperature is reduced, and bacteria and viruses gain a stronger foothold in the low oxygen environment. Individuals suffering from hypoxemia report symptoms like increased headaches, dizziness, insomnia, constipation, faintness, loss of appetite, heart palpitations, impaired kidney functions, cold hands and feet, impaired gland functions and a variety of lymphatic and blood disorders. Oxygen therapies can help bring back the oxygen levels in the body to more normal levels.

I

Immune System: The body's immune system consists of over one trillion white blood cells (lymphocytes) and 100 million molecules called antibodies that are produced and secreted by these lymphocytes. These cells and antibodies find their way into every cell and every space in the body to help protect the body from bacteria, fungi, viruses, parasites, yeasts, molds and even cancer cells during our lifetime. To be "immune" is to be protected, to have resistance, to be exempt from disease. The immune system also includes the skin, which acts as a barrier against disease, the bone marrow, which produces white blood cells, the thymus, spleen, lymph nodes, adenoids and the digestive tract. Oxygen is a key ingredient to a healthy immune system. The lack of oxygen reduces the immune system's ability to fight off disease.

Intracellular Fluid: This is the fluid that is inside every cell. It contains high amounts of potassium, magnesium and phosphate ions and smaller amounts of sodium and chloride ions.

Ion: An electrically charged atom or groups of atoms. Some compounds, like salts, acids and bases, are thought to consist wholly or partly of ions held together by electrical attraction. During the electrolysis process, (a process that is used to make almost all stabilized oxygen solutions today,) negative ions ("anions"), which contain an excess of one or more electrons, and are presented by a negative sign "-" after their chemical symbols, always move towards the anode. The positive ions ("cations"), which are missing one or more electrons, and are represented by a positive sign "+" after their chemical symbols, always move towards the cathode. In gasses, a molecule can lose an electron and become a positive ion and the free electron may attach itself to another molecule or atom and become a negative ion.

Isotope: Any of two or more forms of a chemical element, having the same number of protons in the nucleus, or the same atomic number, but having different numbers of neutrons in the nucleus, or different atomic weights. There are 275 isotopes of the 81 stable elements, in addition to over 800 radioactive isotopes, and every element has known isotopic forms. Isotopes of a single element possess almost identical properties.

K

Kidneys: The kidneys influence and control both body fluids and numerous nutrients that the body requires for metabolism. The kidneys regulate and filter the blood, control electrolytes (like sodium and potassium), regulate the pH of the body to keep the body from becoming too acidic or alkaline, control the amount of water in the body, help eliminate waste products, and produce several very important hormones, especially the ones that help regulate the Production and the release of red blood cells.

Kinesiology: Kinesiology is the scientific study of human or non-human body movement. Kinesiology addresses physiological, biomechanical, and psychological mechanisms of movement. Kinesiology includes the study of orthopedics, strength and conditioning, sport psychology, methods of rehabilitation (physical and occupational therapy), exercise, electrophysiology of muscles and cognitive research techniques.

L

Lactic Acid (2-Hydroxypropanoic acid): Lactic acid is a compound produced when glucose is broken down and oxidized. During intense exercise when oxygen levels are lower, more lactic acid is produced, which can produce hydrogen ions and a burning sensation in muscles while they're active. Despite the myth, however, ongoing soreness in the days following an intense effort is not due to a buildup of lactic acid but tiny muscle tears and inflammations.

Leukocyte (White Blood Cell): A type of blood cell that lacks hemoglobin and is therefore colorless. Leukocytes are capable of ameboid movement. Their chief function is to protect the body against microorganisms causing disease and which may be classified in two main groups: granular and nongranular.

Lipid: Any of a group of organic compounds, including fats, oils, waxes, sterols, and triglycerides, that are insoluble in water, are oily to the touch, and together with carbohydrates and proteins, constitute the principal structural material of living cells.

Liver: The liver is the largest and certainly one of the most important organs in the body. It is our main chemical production factory and has five functions: (1) the production of proteins, including albumin, complement, coagulation factors and globin; (2) the control of glucose by storing extra glucose as glycogen; (3) the control of amino acids; the filtering of poisonous drugs and substances from the blood; (5) the production of bile which carries away wastes and helps in the breakdown and absorption of fats in the small intestine.

Lymphatic (Lymph) System: The liquid volume of the lymphatic system exceeds that of the blood in our bodies. While blood is a carrier of nutrients, lymph actually nourishes the cells. It is designed to filter out of the body large molecules, like bacteria and toxins. Approximately 90% of the fluids in the body pass through the capillaries. The remaining 10%, which includes dead cells and small particles, is transported to the heart through the lymphatic system. This system is remarkable because of its one-way valves called "lymph nodes". These nodes trap micro organisms and foreign bodies. The specialized white blood cells that reside in the nodes (lymphocytes) neutralize and destroy invading pathogens. The lymph constantly circulates through this system. This lymph liquid is moved along by muscle action and not by the pressure created by the pumping of the heart.

Lymphocytes: Lymphocytes are a type of white blood cell that are formed in the lymph glands instead of the bone marrow. These cells travel between the blood stream, lymph glands and the channels between the lymph glands. While there are a number of differentiated lymphocytes, the two most important types are the T-type and the B-type. T-cells are called "killer" white blood cells because they are responsible for attacking abnormal cells in the body, like cancer cells. B-type lymphocytes are responsible for forming antibodies that protect the body against a second attack from diseases that previously found a foothold in the body and that the body was able to defend itself against. These "B-type" cells form an integral part of the immune system.

M

Magnesium: One of the most important minerals in the body and found in over 300 different enzymes that the body uses. It is critically important in the process of creating energy in the cells which involves its combination with glucose and oxygen. Most of the magnesium in the body is used in our bone structure and is actively involved in cellular metabolism. Correct magnesium levels in the body helps protect the body against heart disease, hypoglycemia, reduces kidney stone formation and reduces the severity of P.M.S. A lack of magnesium results in cramping, poor appetite, diarrhea, mental instability, confusion or forgetfulness and even convulsions.

Magnesium Oxide: A molecule in which the mineral magnesium, an essential mineral in the body, is bonded to an oxygen atom forming the chemical combination MgO. Magnesium oxide's molecular bonding, between the magnesium and oxygen atom, can be broken by numerous acids, like citric acid and hydrochloric acid, to release the oxygen molecule for the body to use in its metabolic processes. Magnesium oxide has been used as a body oxygenator.

M.D.R. (Minimum Daily Requirement): Originally, the M.D.R was established by the federal government to prevent acute diseases in animals was promoted during World War II. Today, the Federal Drug Administration (F.D.A.) has established the minimum daily amount of nutrients it recommends to maintain a average health. These minimums include carbohydrates,proteins, etc. (Also see R.D.A.)

Metabolism/Metabolic Cycle: The chemical changes in living cells which provide for the cells' vital process and activities is called the cells' "metabolic cycle". All these functions require the production and use of energy. At the heart of energy production is oxygen An abundance of body oxygen results in excellent energy production and a healthy metabolism. A lack of body oxygen results in poor cellular health, an increase in disease conditions and cellular death.

mg/L (Milligrams per Liter): When dealing with liquids (like water), mg/L = ppm. By definition, a Liter of water weighs 1 kg (1 kilogram or 1000 grams).

Mitochondria: Mitochondria are structures within cells that convert the energy from food into a form that cells can use. Each cell contains hundreds to thousands of mitochondria, which are located in the fluid that surrounds the nucleus (the cytoplasm). Mitochondria produce energy through a process called oxidative phosphorylation. This process uses oxygen and simple sugars to create adenosine triphosphate (ATP), the cell's main energy source.In addition to energy production, mitochondria play a role in several other cellular activities. For example, mitochondria help regulate the self-destruction of cells (apoptosis). They are also necessary for the production of substances such as cholesterol and heme (a component of hemoglobin, the molecule that carries oxygen in the blood).

Molecule: The smallest physical unit of an element or compound, consisting of one or more like atoms in an element and two or more different atoms in a compound.

Monocytes: Monocytes are white blood cells that are similar in function to neutrophils (also called phagocytes). The main difference between these two types of white blood cells is that while in the blood stream, they are the immature precursors to phagocytes. Monocytes do not fully mature until they enter the tissues where they can grow to as much as five times their original size. Monocytes are long-lived white blood cells, residing in the tissues from several months to as long as seven years, performing their specific protective functions.

Myofibril: One of the fine longitudinal fibrils in the skeletal or cardiac (heart) muscle fibers that is made up of many regularly overlapped ultramicroscopic thick and thin myofiliments.

Myofilament: A myofilament is a chain of protein molecules found in the myofibrils of a striated muscle. There are two types of myofilament, thin and thick, with the thin filaments being made primarily of the protein actin and the thick ones primarily comprised of the protein myosin. In striated muscle tissue, the filaments are arranged within the myofibrils in repeating polypeptide complexes called sarcomeres. The protein molecules play an important role in muscle contraction and relaxation. Striated muscle is found throughout the body in the form of skeletal muscle, which is a type of muscle whose contractions and movements can be consciously controlled. Cardiac muscle is also striated, and is found only within the walls of the heart. Within the cells of striated muscles are tubular organelles called myofibrils. The myofibrils are made up of bundles of protein in the form of thick and thin myofilaments. In striated muscle tissue, a myofilament has a set length that doesn't change, even when the muscle shortens as it contracts or elongates as it relaxes again. A thin myofilament is primarily made of a protein called actin, which assembles itself into a ladder-like scaffold during muscle contraction that the myosin filaments can then use to generate force.

Myosin: A protein that binds with actin filaments and helps in the contraction of myofibrils in muscle cells.

N

Naturopathy: Naturopathy is believed to be the oldest form of practicing medicine. The term is derived from the Greek word "natura", meaning "nature", and "pathos", meaning suffering. Combined together, the word means "nature is used to heal". Naturopathy is a system, practice or science using natural remedies to heal instead of synthetic drugs, surgeries or non-natural medical practices.

Neutron: A neutron is a very small particle of matter that has no electrical charge and is part of the nucleus of all atoms except hydrogen atoms.

Neutrophils: Neutrophils are white blood cells that are responsible for isolating and killing bacteria that have invaded the body. Also called "phagocytes" (which means to "engulf',) these cells actually surround and swallow bacteria in the blood stream. Though neutrophils' life spans are short, usually just a few days, they are powerful and strategic hunters supporting the immune system.

O

Obligate anaerobe: An organism that can grow only in the complete absence of molecular oxygen.

Organelles: Specialized structures in every cell which include mitochondria, Golgi apparatus, centrioles, granular and agranular endoplasmic reticulum, nucleus, DNA, proteins, vacuoles, microsomes, lysosomes, plasma membrane and fibrils.

ORP (Oxidation-Reduction Potential): Oxidation-reduction potential, or ORP, is a measurement that indicates the degree to which a substance is capable of oxidizing or reducing another substance. ORP is measured in millivolts (mv) using an ORP meter. A positive ORP reading indicates that a substance is an oxidizing agent. The higher the reading, the more oxidizing it is. As such, a substance with an ORP reading of +400 mv is 4 times more oxidizing than a substance with an ORP reading of +100 mv. A negative ORP reading indicates that a substance is a reducing agent. The lower the reading, the more anti-oxidizing it is. As such, a substance with an ORP reading of -400 mv is 4 times more anti-oxidizing than a substance with an ORP reading of -100 mv.

Oxidation: The process by which an atom or molecule is changed electrically by the addition or subtraction of electrons altering the electrochemical makeup and function of the original atom or molecule. At the center of all oxidation processes are oxygen atoms. Burning is an example of rapid oxidation; rusting is an example of slow oxidation.

Oxidative Stress: A term used to describe the effect of oxidation in which an abnormal level of reactive oxygen species (ROS), such as the free radicals (hydroxyl, nitric acid, superoxide) or the non-radicals (hydrogen peroxide, lipid peroxide) lead to damage (called oxidative damage) to specific molecules with consequential injury to cells or tissue.

Oxygen: The most important element for all life. Named by its discoverer Lavoisier from the Greek word "oxygene" meaning "acid" and "gignesthai" meaning "to be born" since he believed that oxygen was the prime ingredient in all acids. Oxygen is a colorless, tasteless gas that comprises as much as 23% of our atmosphere. Oxygen is a critical ingredient in the oxidation of glucose in the cells to form energy. Oxygen is the most abundant of all the elements and combines chemically with more elements than any other. It is the largest component of organic molecules and is crucial in the respiratory process of animals.

Oxygen Consumption (VO_2): VO_2 (or oxygen consumption) is a measure of the volume of oxygen that is used by your body to convert the energy from the food you eat into the energy molecules, called adenosine triphosphate (ATP), that the body uses at the cellular level.

Oxygen Delivery (DO_2): DO_2 is the supply of oxygen per unit of time to a tissue, organ or the entire body.

Oxygen Demand: Oxygen demand is a a theoretical concept describing the amount of oxygen that a tissue, organ or entire patient would need to consume to meet all of its needs under a given set of circumstances. Oxygen demand cannot be measured, but it is a useful concept when reflecting upon the factors that affect oxygen delivery and consumption.

Oxygen Starvation: The physiological condition where the body lacks a sufficient supply of oxygen for normal cellular functions. The result is a drastic pH (acid-alkaline) change, poor metabolic functioning, an increase in body toxins and subsequent fatigue, illness, disease and even death.

Oxygen Therapies: Any modality which introduces oxygen and related therapies as part of a health regimen. These therapies can include deep breathing exercises, hydrogen peroxide and oxidative therapies, ozone therapies, hyperbaric oxygen therapies, ionization therapies and the ingestion of oral stabilized oxygen products. Oxygen therapies are considered an alternative approach to health.

Ozone: An allotropic (different) form of oxygen containing three oxygen atoms (O-O-O or O_3). Ozone comes from the Greek word "ozein" which means "to smell" since ozone has a distinctive and peculiar odor which is similar to the smell of chlorine. Ozone is a very active oxidizing agent and reacts with many other atoms, molecules and compounds. It is also an excellent deodorizer and disinfectant that kills most known pathogenic organisms.

P

PaO$_2$: The partial pressure of oxygen in arterial blood, arterial oxygen concentration, or tension. PaO$_2$ is usually expressed in millimeters of mercury (mm/Hg).

Pathogens (Pathogenic): An organism that causes disease. Pathogenic organisms include viruses, bacteria, yeasts, molds, fungi and parasites. These organisms use the body as the host to provide them with favorable conditions to multiply. The toxins excreted by these organisms, or their consumption of vital nutrients that they require to grow and reproduce, taxes the body's immune system and reduces the body's oxygen levels and thus the body's ability to fight off these invading pathogens.

pH: A chemistry term that denotes the negative logarithm of the concentration of hydrogen ions in gram atoms in a liter of solution. pH is used to express acidity or alkalinity of a solution or material. pH values range from "0" to "14" with "7" representing neutral pH. Numbers less than seven in value are considered acidic and numbers above seven are considered alkaline. The low pH and high pH values indicate substances that could be caustic and thus toxic to the human body.

Phagocytosis: Phagocytosis is a type of endocytosis. Endocytosis is a process in which a cell absorbs a particle, molecule, bacterium, or other type of matter by engulfing it. Phagocytosis refers to the engulfing of larger, solid particles. Often the engulfed particle is another cell, like when a white blood cell, which is a part of the immune system, engulfs a bacterium to destroy it.

Plasma (Blood Plasma): The almost clear liquid component of blood that is 95% water. The remaining 5% is dissolved nutrients, waste products from cellular metabolism, proteins and hormones. The nutrients include sugars, fats amino acids, vitamins and minerals.

Platelets: Platelets are special cells in the blood stream that help stop bleeding and also repair damaged blood vessels by sticking to the vessel walls and adhering to each other to form a dam-like structure.

Platelets are also called blood platelets or thrombocytes.

PPM (Parts per Million): Just as percent means out of a hundred, so parts per million or ppm means out of a million. PPM usually describes the concentration of something in water or soil. One ppm is equivalent to 1 milligram of something per liter of water (mg/l) or 1 milligram of something per kilogram soil (mg/kg).

Potassium: Along with calcium and magnesium, potassium plays a major part in maintaining cardiovascular health. Potassium works hand-in-hand with sodium in what is called the "potassium pump", an action that transfers nutrients and oxygen into the cells and removes wastes and carbon dioxide out of the cells. Potassium lowers blood pressure and reduces the possibility of strokes. A lack of potassium can result in higher blood pressure, edema (excess water) in the tissues and a more rapid heart rate.

Proteins: Proteins are naturally occurring combinations of amino acids which contain carbon, hydrogen, nitrogen, oxygen and usually sulphur. Proteins are the most important constituents of all living cells and a crucial part of the diet of all higher life forms. There are two main types of proteins: (1) fibrous, which are insoluble and form the structural foundations of our hair, skin, tendons, cartilage and muscles; (2) globular proteins, which are soluble and include enzymes, hormones, hemoglobin and antibodies.

Proton: A positively charged elementary particle that is a fundamental constituent of all atomic nuclei. It is the lightest and most stable baryon, having a charge equal in magnitude to that of the electron, a spin of ½, and a mass of 1.673×10^{-27} kg. Symbol: P.

Protoplasm: See "Cytoplasm".

Q

Quantum (theory, mechanics): Theory of physics that explains the behavior of nature and its forces on a very small, subatomic scale. The theory states that physical quantities can only have discrete values (this is quantization). According to quantum mechanics photons or electrons may be considered as particles but they can also be diffracted like waves (this is referred to as wave-particle duality). This quantum theory was proposed by Max Planck in 1900. Quantum mechanics is the more formal mathematical description of his theory which was developed in the 1920's. It also incorporates the uncertainty principle, which states that you cannot measure a particle's position and velocity at the same time. The more accurately you know its position, the less accurately you know its velocity and vice versa.

Quantum State: A description in quantum mechanics of a physical system or part of a physical system. Different quantum states for a physical system show discrete differences in the value of the variables used to define the state. For example, the spin of an isolated electron can take on one of only two values; there are no other quantum states available for the electron and no intermediate values, since spin is quantized. The quantum state is sometimes described by a set of quantum numbers that pick out the appropriate values for describing the state.

Quark: An elementary particle which is believed to be the fundamental structural unit from which all other particles are made. There are six quarks: up, down, strange, charm, top and bottom. A proton is made up of one down quark and two up quarks.

R

Radiation Therapy: A cancer therapy where X-rays or other rays that produce ionizing radiation are focused on cancer cells. As this radiation passes through living and healthy tissue, it slows the tissue's development or destroys the tissue altogether. The effects of exposure to radiation depends on the dosage, the time of exposure (length) and the duration (number of days, weeks, months) of the treatment. Radiation therapy may produce very unpleasant side effects (called radiation sickness) including fatigue, nausea, loss of appetite and vomiting. Radiation therapy kills both healthy and unhealthy cells. Radiation is not selective.

Reactive Oxygen Species (ROS): Molecules and ions of oxygen that have an unpaired electron making them extremely reactive. Many cellular structures are susceptible to attack by ROS which has been linked as a cause of cancer, heart disease, and cerebrovascular disease.

Recommended Daily Allowance: R.D.A., also called the U.S.R.D.A., is a listing of vitamins and minerals that the Federal Drug Association has established as the level necessary to maintain average health and to prevent nutritional deficiency. These amounts are as follows:

Vitamin A	5,000 IU
Vitamin C	60 mg

Calcium	1,000 mg	Pantothenic Acid	10 mg
Iron	19 mg	Phosphorus	1,000 mg
Vitamin D	400 IU	Iodine	150 mcg
Vitamin E	30 IU	Magnesium	400 mg
Vitamin K	80 mcg	Zinc	15 mg
Thiamin (B1)	1.5 mg	Selenium	70 mcg
Riboflavin (B2)	1.7 mg	Copper	2 mg
Niacin (B3)	20 mg	Manganese	2 mg
Vitamin B	62 mg	Chromium	120 mcg
Vitamin B12	6 mcg	Molybdenum	75 mcg
Folate (Folic Acid)	400 mcg	Chloride	3,400 mg
Biotin	300 mcg		

Recovery: The Recovery Principle dictates that athletes need adequate time to recuperate from training and competition. Many believe that an athlete's ability to recover from workouts is just as important as the workout itself. It is during rest periods that athletes' bodies adapt to the stress placed upon them during intense workout sessions and competitions. Rest also provides time for a mental preparation and reflection. The Recovery Principle applies both to immediate rest needed between bouts of exercise, as well as to longer time intervals of several hours to about two days.

Red Blood Cells: Doughnut-shaped cells in the plasma whose main purpose is to transport oxygen to the cells of the body and remove carbon dioxide from the same cells. Red blood cells contain the protein hemoglobin which has the remarkable chemical ability to hold oxygen captive while the cell traverses the thousands of miles of arteries and capillaries in the body.

Reduction: A chemical reaction in which an atom or ion gains electrons, thus undergoing a decrease in valence. If an iron atom having a valence of $+3$ gains an electron, the valence decreases to $+2$.

Respiration: Respiration is a process which provides body with oxygen for growth and other metabolic activities and removes waste products in the form of carbon dioxide gas. The exchange of gases take place in the Lungs. The Lungs are the main organs involved in the respiration process. Air passes into the lungs through the process of inhalation through the nostrils and the air flows down the trachea into the lungs. The Lungs have alveoli which are small air sacs and is filled with tiny capillaries which are functional in the carrying of oxygen and carbon dioxide back and forth from the heart to the lungs. Within the cells, respiration is a process where carbohydrates, mainly as glucose, is broken down and energy (ATP) is released. This energy is used by the cells for various functions and processes from muscle contraction to cell building, repair and growth.

S

Sarcolemma: The thin membrane enclosing a striated muscle fiber.

Sarcomere: The structural unit of a striped muscle fiber. (See Myofibril.)

Singlet Oxygen: An excited or higher-energy form of oxygen characterized by the spin of a pair of electrons in opposite directions. The electron spin is unidirectional (same direction)in normal molecular oxygen It is an extremely reactive form of oxygen. Although it exists for no more than 0.1 second, it may react with atmospheric pollutants to foster smog formation and may have harmful biological effects.

Sodium: One of the essential minerals needed for a healthy body. Sodium plays a strategic role, along with potassium, in moving nutrients and oxygen into the cells and removing waste products and carbon dioxide out of the cell in an ionic pumping action. Contrary to the belief that high concentrations of sodium cause high blood pressure, there appears to be more medical evidence indicating that a deficiency in potassium, not too much sodium, may be the primary cause of this condition.

Stabilized Oxygen: Stabilized oxygen is a classification of allotropic forms of oxygen that are combined with other atoms that enables the oxygen to become electrically stable in its attachment to the new molecule. Once in this "stable" state, this new compound can be used as a delivery source for the oxygen as a dietary supplement. These stabilized oxygen molecules may be both in a liquid or dry form. Types of stabilized oxygen include hydrogen peroxide (food grade), chlorine dioxide (chlorite), magnesium peroxide, chlorate and the dissolved diatomic (O_2) oxygen found in a small number of products.

Stamina: Stamina is staying power or enduring strength. Stamina is not always related to physical strength and endurance. Solving a difficult puzzle or a complex problem requires your brain to work long and hard, something called mental stamina.

Sugars: Sugar is one of the two key elements needed for the production of energy in every cell. (The other is oxygen.) Cells derive the sugar they need for "combustion" in creating A.T.P. energy from breaking down carbohydrates into the simplest form of sugar, glucose.

Superoxide: A common reactive form of oxygen (O_2^-) that is formed when molecular oxygen gains a single electron. Superoxide radicals can attack susceptible biological targets, including lipids, proteins, and nucleic acids. It is aN intermediate in numerous biological oxidations and an important killing mechanism generated in lysosomes of phagocytes after they have phagocytosed microorganisms.

Superoxide Dismutase: Superoxide Dismutase (SOD) is metal-containing antioxidant enzyme that reduces potentially harmful free radicals of oxygen formed during normal metabolic cell processes to oxygen and hydrogen peroxide.

Sympathetic nerve: A nerve of the autonomic nervous system that regulates involuntary and automatic reactions, especially to stress.

T

TDS (Total Dissolved Solids): TDS refers to any minerals, salts, metals, cations or anions dissolved in water. Total dissolved solids include inorganic salts, (principally calcium, magnesium, potassium, sodium, bicarbonates, chlorides, and sulfates,) and small amounts of organic matter that are dissolved in water.

Tendons and Ligaments: A tendon connects muscle to bone, while a ligament connects two bones. Tendons let your muscles move bones, whereas ligaments stabilize joints. Both tendons and ligaments are fibrous tissues designed to connect parts of your body. This tissue is tougher and less flexible for tendons and stringier and more elastic for ligaments. However, both tendons and ligaments require some degree of flexibility to accommodate movement; rigid tendons and ligaments would prevent basic body movements. When tendons and ligaments are stretched beyond their basic capacity, they become damaged. For tendons, this can result in tendonitis, which occurs when the tendon becomes torn. This damage causes the tissue of the tendon to inflame while it heals; as a result, tendonitis causes swelling and soreness, as well as temporary loss of muscle function. Ligaments also suffer damage when stretched beyond their limits. As with tendons, this can result in tears of the tissue. Ligament tears weaken the joint and threaten its integrity.

Tetraoxygen (O_4): An allotrope of oxygen having four atoms in each molecule instead of the normal two.

Trace Mineral (Essential): Minerals that are essential for maintaining optimum health but are not required in large quantities are called essential trace minerals. There are dozens of trace minerals that are important in small amounts to insure normal functioning of metabolism and the immune system.

V

Valence: A whole number that represents the ability of an atom or a group of atoms to combine with other atoms or groups of atoms. The valence is determined by the number of electrons that an atom can lose, add, or share. An atom's valence is positive if its own electrons are used in forming the bond, or negative if another atom's electrons are used. For example, a carbon atom can share four of its electrons with other atoms and therefore has a valence of $^{+}4$. A sodium atom can receive an electron from another atom and therefore has a valence of $^{-}1$. The valence of an atom generally indicates how many chemical bonds it is capable of forming with other atoms. Also called valence number or oxidation state.

Veins, Arteries and Capillaries (Blood Vessels): There are three types of blood vessels, each with its own function. Veins carry blood back to the heart, arteries carry blood away from the heart and capillaries connect arteries to veins. Thin and weak, capillaries are only as thick as one epithelial cell. Blood passes through capillaries one cell at a time, single file. The blood cells release oxygen, which passes through the capillary walls into nearby tissue. Tissues then release carbon dioxide through the capillary walls which are picked up by the red blood cells.

Virus: Some have described a virus as a living crystal that changes its form. A virus, as opposed to a bacteria, lives out its life cycle within the cell by invading the cell and changing the cell's DNA to replicate the virus. For this reason it is more difficult to "kill" viruses with traditional drugs and therapies because a virus resides inside the cell emerging only when the cell bursts and the new viruses invade new cells to reproduce once again. Oxygen appears to be the only totally effective defense against a virus infection.

Vitamins: Vitamins are essential compounds that the body must have for normal cellular metabolism. With few exceptions, (like Vitamin D, for example,) vitamins cannot be manufactured by the body and must be derived from the foods we eat. There are 13 major vitamins in two categories: (1) fat soluble and (2) water soluble. The fat soluble vitamins, like A, D, E and K, come directly from foods that contain fats. These vitamins are absorbed into the blood stream in the intestines and then stored in fatty tissue (like the liver) until the body needs them. These vitamins are stored and not excreted or eliminated from the body. Water soluble vitamins, like C, B12, Bl, B2, B6, panthothenic acid, biotin and folic acid, are derived from vegetables and fruits and are not stored in the body. They must be supplied on a daily basis. Any excesses of these vitamins are excreted by the body.

VO$_2$: See "Oxygen Consumption".

W

White Blood Cells: The principle role of the white blood cell is to act as the first line of defense for the immune system against infectious organisms that enter the body. These remarkable soldiers fall into three main categories: (1) granulocytes (which include neutrophils, basophils and eosinophils,) (2) monocytes, and (3) lymphocytes (which include T-type and B-Type cells.) Also see "Leukocytes".

Wild Type (WT): Wild Type is a term referring to the natural genetic form of an organism. A Wild Type is distinguished from a mutant form (an organism with a genetic mutation) and is based on a single mutation. Within the population of an organism, there is no such thing as a wild type. The term, however, is useful for geneticists because it allows a simple definition of a standard or control condition.

X

X-chromosome: One of two sex chromosomes in higher organisms that defines the gender of the adult. In almost all sexually reproducing organisms, the X-chromosome defines female characteristics.

Xenobiotics: The term xenobiotics is used to describe a foreign particle or molecule that is potentially dangerous or toxic.

Y

Y-chromosome: One of two sex chromosomes in higher organisms that defines the gender of the adult. In almost all sexually reproducing organisms, the Y-chromosome defines male characteristics.

Yeast: Yeast is a class of minute, uni-cellular fungi that function either aerobically or anaerobically within the body. The most serious pathogenic yeast is Candida albicans (see "Candida") which resides in the digestive tract. Normally kept under control by a beneficial microorganism, Acidophilus, Candida can spread whenever the body is low on oxygen, where the body has too high of a level of stored sugars or when the acid balance of the body has been thrown off because of diet or disease. Candida infections can cause bloating, diarrhea, constipation, burning, gas and cramping. Candida can invade the entire body not just the intestinal and urinary tract.

APPENDIX TWO:
For Further Study:
Articles and Research to satisfy your hunger for more information:

Some of the following articles may be older but the information is as accurate today as it was several decades ago. Sadly, we live in a new generation that experiences "lost information syndrome" because the focus is on instant "new" quick "tweets" that overshadow more historical research from the past.

For the most complete listing of articles on oxygen therapies, ozone and hydrogen peroxide, contact Dr. Gene Meyer, D.D.S. A biochemist, who has devoted much of his professional life to the study of oxygen and its effects on disease, Dr. Meyer has amassed one of the largest collections of oxygen-based literature in the U.S. today, almost 10,000 articles. His address is: 9725 E. Flower Street, Bellflower, CA 90706.

Priestley, Joseph, LL.D.F.R.S. Experiments and Observations on Different Kinds of Air and Other Branches of Natural Philosophy Connected with the Subject (in three volumes). Printed by Thomas Pearson and Sold by J. Johnson, St. Paul's Church-Yard, London. MDCCXC.

"The oxygen crisis: Could the decline of oxygen in the atmosphere undermine our health and threaten human survival?"
Peter Tatchell, guardian.co.uk 13 August 2008.
http://www.guardian.co.uk/commentisfree/2008/aug/13/carbonemissions.climatechange

"How fast does blood travel through the normal human body?"
http://answers.yahoo.com/question/index?qid=20081203093048AAeITP8

"High dose of oxygen enhances natural cancer treatment"
Hannah Hickey, April 4, 2011
http://www.washington.edu/news/articles/high-dose-of-oxygen-enhances-natural-cancer-treatment

"Oxygen regulation and limitation to cellular respiration in mouse skeletal muscle in vivo"
David J. Marcinek, Wayne A. Ciesielski, Kevin E. Conley and Kenneth A. Schenkman

Departments of Radiology, Physiology and Biophysics and Bioengineering, and Pediatrics, Anesthesiology, and Bioengineering, University of Washington Medical Center, Seattle 98195; and Children's Hospital and Regional Medical Center, Seattle, Washington 98105, Submitted 11 March 2003
http://ajpheart.physiology.org/content/285/5/H1900.abstract

"What is the Immune System?"
U.S. Department of Health and Human Services
National Institute of Health
http://www.niaid.nih.gov/topics/immuneSystem/pages/whatisimmunesystem.aspx

The Oxygen Revolution: Hyperbaric Oxygen Therapy: The Groundbreaking New Treatment for Stroke, Alzheimer's, Parkinson's, Arthritis, Autism, Learning Disabilities and More
2010 Updated Edition Hatherleigh Press (April 24, 2007)
Paul G. Harch (Author), Virginia McCullough (Author)

"The Surgical Uses of Ozone". Stoker, George. Lancet II, October 21, 1916, page 712.
http://www.musa-group.com/premotes/stoker1916.pdf.

The FDA Continues to Suppress Ozone Therapy Despite Proven Efficacy
February 19, 2010, Paul Fassa
http://www.naturalnews.com/028201_ozone_therapy_FDA.html#ixzz1YAE9d4bk

FDA to Ban Food Nutrients
September 16, 2011,Staff Report, The Daily Bell
http://www.thedailybell.com/2941/FDA-to-Ban-Food-Nutrients

Evolution of Oxygen Utilization in Multicellular Organisms and Implications for Cell Signaling in Tissue Engineering.
Stamati, Katerina, Vivek Mudera, and Umber Cheema. Journal of Tissue Engineering 2.1 (2011): 2041731411432365. PMC. Web. 29 Feb. 2016.

"Oxygen and Life on Earth."
Lindahl, Sten G. E. Anesthesiology 109.1 (2008): 7-13.

Understanding the Two Sides of Oxygen. Cracking the Metabolic Code: The Nine Keys to Peak Health and Longevity.
LaValle, James B. Chapter 15. North Bergen, NJ: Basic Health, 2003. 373.

"Bio-Oxidative Therapy".
Altman, Nathaniel. Natural Health, November/December 1995:44.

"Environmental and Physical Stress and Nutrient Requirements."
Askew, Dr. Eldon W., Ph.D. American Journal of Clinical Nutrition, 1995;61 (Suppl.): 631S-7S. American Society for Clinical Nutrition.

Freedom from Disease: How to Control Free Radicals. Ayur-Ved, Maharishi. Veda Publishing, Toronto, Canada: 1993.

"Keep Breathing".
Baranowski, Zane. Health Freedom News, October 1988: 31-34.

'The Role of Active Oxygen in Microbial Killing by Phagocytes."

Babior, B.M., 1982: Pathology of Oxygen, New York: Academic Press.

"Technical Discussion: Stabilized Oxygen."
Berg, Dr. James O., Ph.D. Search For Health (U.S.A.), 1988.

"Age of the Virus".
Bland, Jeffrey S., Ph.D. Delicious, November 1993:40-43.

Oxidology: The Study of Reactive Oxygen Toxic Species (ROTS) and their Metabolism in Health and Disease."
Bradford, R.W., Allen, H.W. and Culbert, M.L. The Robert W. Bradford Foundation, A Trust, Los Altos, CA (1985).

"Health Effects of Alternative Disinfectants and Their Reaction Products,"
Bull, R.J.,J. AWWA, May: 229 (1980).

"Toxicological Problems Associated with Alternative Methods of Disinfection,"
Bull, R.J., J. AWWA Dec: 642 (1982).

"Are You Overdoing Antioxidants?"
Challem, Jack. Natural Health, May/June 1995.

"Free Radicals and Antioxidants: A Contrarian View?" Challem, Jack. Nutrition Review, Natural Food Merchandiser Nutrition Science News, December 1995.

"Inside Out."
Gchoke, Dr. Anthony, M.A., D.C., D.A.C.B.N. The Energy Times, July I August 1994.

The Unsung Antioxidant: Zinc.
Gchoke, Dr. Anthony, M.A., D.C., D.A.C.B.N. "Total Health", December 1993.

Oxygen - Oxygen - Oxygen
Donsbach, Kurt, N.D., Ph.D. Rockland Corporation: 1993; 13.

"Dinosaurs Weren't Done In By Asteroids"
Associated Press Release, October 27, 1997.

"Antibiotics: Too Much of a Good Thing?"
Finn, Kathleen, Delicious, October 1995: 30-34.

"Confessions of an Herbalist: The Magic of Aerobic Oxygen"
Goulet, Brian. Focus on Nutrition - The Canadian Journal of Health & Nutrition. (Issue No. 21), Burnaby, BC, 1989, Academic Press, N. Y., 1977.

"Hyperbaric Oxygen Therapy"
Grim, Pamela, Lawrence Gottlieb, Allyn Boddie and Eric Batson. Journal of the American Medical Association, April 25, 1990, V. 263, n16: 2216(5).

The Textbook of Medical Physiology, (5th Edition)
Guyton, Arthur C. Pennsylvania:WB Saunders Co., 1976.

"Reactive oxygen species in living systems: source, biochemistry, and role in human disease."
Halliwell, Dr. Barry, Ph.D. American Journal of Medicine, September 30, 1991, v91n3C p145(9).

International Association for Oxygen Therapy.
A Division of American Society of Medical Missionaries. P.O. Box 1360, Priest River, ID 83856. (208) 448-2657.

"Antioxidant Adaptation: It's Role in Free Radical Pathology."
Levine, Dr. Stephen and Kidd, Dr. Parris. Biocurrents Press, San Francisco, 1987.

"Beyond Anti-Oxidant Adaptation: A Free Radical-Hypoxia-Oonal Thesis of Cancer Causation,"
Levine, Dr. Stephen and Kidd, Dr. Parris. 1985, J. Orthomol. Medicine, 14(3):189-213.

"Immunity, Cancer, Oxygen, and Candida Albicans". Let's Live, August, 1986.

Medicine at the Crossroads
Logan, Cordell, Ph.D., N.D. Logan Press, Logan, UT (1993)

"Safety of Oral Chlorine Dioxide, Chlorite, and Chlorate Ingestion in Man."
Lubbers,J.R., J.R. Bianchine, and R.J. Bull. Ch. 95,pp 1335-1341 in R.L. Jolley, Ed. Water Chlorination: Environmental Impact and Health Effects, Vol. 4 Ann Arbor Science, Ann Arbor, MI (1982).

Oxygen Therapies: A New Way of Approaching Diseases.
McCabe, Ed. Energy Publications, Morrisville, NY (1994).

Superoxides and Superoxide Dismutases.
McCord, Joe and Findivich, Irwin. Academic Press, N. Y., 1977.

"Hazards of Hypoxemia,"
McGaffigan, Patricia A., R.N., M.S. Nursing, May, 1996.

Chlorine Dioxide: Chemistry and Environmental Impact of Oxychlorine Compounds.
Masschelein, W.J. and Rice, Rip G. Ann Arbor Science Publishers, Inc.,Ann Arbor, MI.

"The case for Stabilized Oxygen".
Muntz, John, D.O., Ph.D. Health World, August 1991: 12.

"Ozone Selectivity Inhibits the Growth of Human Cancer Cells."
Sweet, F. et al. Science: 209:931(1980)

"Oxygen -O2: The Life Giving Element."
Starr, Sonya C., B.S., N.C. The Nutrition & Dietary Consultant, August 1986.

"Drugs, Not Foods, Are Toxic."
Sevy, Jonathan B., D.C. Dynamic Chiropractic. December 17, 1993.

"Invisible Toxins Hurt the Immune System."
Thompson, Donald C., M.D. Journal of Longevity Research, Vol3, No. 5, 1997:26-27.

"Why antibiotics are failing to protect us from seemingly common viruses and what you can do to protect yourself."
Energy Times, March 1996: 29-33.

APPENDIX THREE:
On the Origin of Cancer Cells

Dr. Otto Warburg, Ph.D.[196]

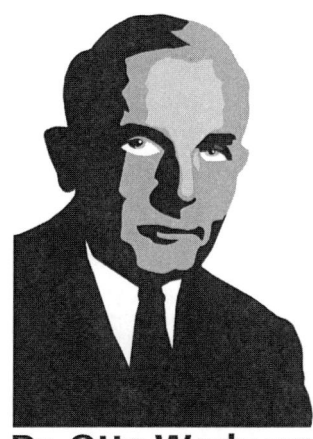

Dr. Otto Warburg

Our principal experimental object for the measurement of the metabolism of cancer cells is today no longer the tumor, but the ascites cancer cells (1) living free in the abdominal cavity, which are almost pure cultures of cancer cells with which one can work quantitatively as in chemical analysis. Formerly it could be said of tumors, with their varying cancer cell content, that they ferment more strongly the more cancer cells they contain, but today we can determine the absolute fermentation values of the cancer cells and find such high values that we come very close to the fermentation values of wildly proliferating Torula yeasts.

What was formerly only qualitative has now become quantitative. What was formerly only probable has now become certain. The era in which the fermentation of the cancer cells or its importance could be disputed is over, and no one today can doubt that we understand the origin of cancer cells if we know how their large fermentation originates, or, to express it more fully,

---

[196] Professor Otto Warburg was the director of the Max Planck Institute for Cell Physiology, Berlin-Dahlem, Germany. This paper is based on a lecture delivered at Stuttgart on May 25, 1955, before the German Central Committee for Cancer Control. It was first published in German {Naturwissenschaften 42, 401 (1955)}1. This translation was prepared by Dean Burk, Jehu Hunter, and W.Wh. Everhardy of the United States Department of Health, Education, and Welfare, Public Health Service, National Institutes of Health, Bethesda, Maryland, with permission of Naturwissenschaften and with collaboration of Professor Warburg, who introduced additional material. Published in SCIENCE, February 4, 1956, Volume 13, Number 3191, pp. 309-314

if we know how the damaged respiration and the excessive fermentation of the cancer cells originate.

We now understand the chemical mechanisms of respiration and fermentation almost completely, but we do not need this knowledge for what follows, since energy alone will be the center of our consideration. We need to know no more of respiration and fermentation here than that they are energy-producing re actions and that they synthesize the energy-rich adenosine triphosphate (A.T.P.), through which the energy of respiration and fermentation is then made available for life.

Since it is known how much adenosine triphosphate can be synthesized by respiration and how much by fermentation, we can write immediately the potential, biologically utilizable energy production of any cells if we have measure their respiration and fermentation rates. With the ascites cancer cells of the mouse, for example, we find an average respiration rate of seven cubic millimeters of oxygen consumed per milligram, per hour, and a fermentation rate of 60 cubic millimeters of lactic acid produced per milligram, per hour. This, converted to energy equivalents, means that the cancer cells can obtain approximately the same amount of energy from fermentation as from respiration, whereas the normal body cells obtain much more energy from respiration than from fermentation. For example, the liver and the kidney of an adult animal obtain about 100 times as much energy from respiration as from fermentation.

I shall not consider aerobic fermentation, which is a result of the interaction of respiration and fermentation, because aerobic fermentation is too labile and too dependent on external conditions. Of importance for the considerations that follow are only the two stable independent metabolic processes, respiration and anaerobic fermentation: respiration, which is measured by the oxygen consumption of cells that are saturated with oxygen; and fermentation, which is measured by the formation of lactic acid in the absence of oxygen.

Since the respiration of all cancer cells is damaged, our firm question is, "How can the respiration of body cells be injured?" Of this damage to respiration, it can be said at the outset that it must be irreversible, since the respiration of cancer cells can never return to normal.

Second, the injury to respiration must not be so great that the cells are killed, for then no cancer cells could result. If respiration is damaged when it forms too little adenosine triphosphate, it may be either that the oxygen consumption has been decreased or that, with undiminished oxygen consumption, the coupling between respiration and the formation of adenosine triphosphate has been broken, as was first pointed out by Feodor Lynen (2).

One method for the destruction of the respiration of body cells is removal of oxygen. If, for example, embryonal tissue is exposed to an oxygen deficiency for some hours, and then is placed in oxygen again, 50 percent more of the respiration is destroyed.

The cause of this destruction of respiration is lack of energy. As a matter of fact, the cells need their respiratory energy to preserve their structure, and if respiration is inhibited, both structure and respiration disappear.

Another method for destroying respiration is to use respiratory poisons. From the standpoint of energy, this method comes to the same result as the first method. No matter whether oxygen is withdrawn from the cell or whether the oxygen is prevented from reacting by a poison, the result is the same in both cases-namely, impairment of respiration from lack of energy.

I may mention a few respiratory poisons. A strong, specific respiratory poison is arsenious acid, which as every clinician knows, may produce cancer. Hydrogen sulfide and many of its derivatives are also strong, specific respiratory poisons. We know today that certain hydrogen sulfide derivatives, thiourea and thioacetamide, with which citrus fruit juices have been preserved in recent times, induce cancer of the liver and gall bladder in rats.

Urethane is a nonspecific respiratory poison. It inhibits respiration as a chemically indifferent narcotic, since it displaces metabolites from cell structures. In recent years, it has been recognized that sub-narcotic doses of urethane cause lung cancer in mice in 100 percent of treatments. Urethane is particularly suitable as a carcinogen, because in contrast to alcohol, it is not itself burned up on the respiring surfaces, and, unlike ether or chloroform, it does not cytolize the cells. Any narcotic that has these proper ties may cause cancer upon chronic administration in small doses.

The first notable experimental induction of cancer by oxygen deficiency was described by Goldblatt and Cameron (3), who exposed heart fibroblasts in tissue culture to intermittent oxygen deficiency for long periods, and finally obtained transplantable cancer cells, whereas in control cultures that were maintained without oxygen deficiency, no cancer cells resulted. clinical experiences along these lines are innumerable: the production of cancer by intermittent irritation of the outer skin and of the mucosa of internal organs, by the plugging of the excretory ducts of glands, by cirrhoses of tissues, and so forth. In all these cases, the intermittent irritation lead to intermittent circulatory disturbances. Probably chronic intermittent oxygen deficiency plays a greater role in the formation of cancer in the body than does the chronic administration of respiratory poisons.

Any respiratory injury due to lack of energy, however, whether it is produced by oxygen deficiency or by respiratory poisons, must be cumulative, since it is irreversible. Frequent, small doses of respiratory poisons are therefore more dangerous than a single large dose, where there is al ways the chance that the cells will be killed rather than that they will become carcinogenic.

If an injury of respiration is to produce cancer, this injury must, as already mention, be irreversible. We understand by this not only that the inhibition of respiration remains after removal of the respiratory poison, but, even more, that the inhibition of respiration also continues through all the following cell division, for measurements of metabolism in transplanted tumors have shown that cancer cells cannot regain normal respiration, even in the course of many decades, once they have lost it.

This originally mysterious phenomenon has been ex plained by a discovery that comes from the early years of cell physiology (4). When liver cells were cytolized by infusion of water and the cytolyzate was centrifuged, it was found that the greater part of the respiration sank to the bottom with the cell grana.

It was also shown that the respiration of the centrifuged grana was inhibited by narcotics at concentrations affecting cell structures, from which it was concluded - already in 1914- that the respiring grana are not insoluble cell particles but autonomous organisms, a result that has been extended in recent years by the English botanist Darlington (5) and particularly by Mark Woods and H.G. du Buy (6) of the National Cancer Institute in Bethesda, Maryland.

Woods and du Buy have experimentally expanded our concepts concerning the self-perpetuating nature of mitochondrial elements (grana) and have demonstrated the hereditary role of extranuclear aberrant forms of these in the causation of neoplasia. The autonomy of the respiring grana, both biochemically and genetically, can hardly be doubted today.

If the principle "Omne granum e grano" is valid for respiring grana, we understand why the respiration connected with grana remains damaged when it has once been damaged; it is for the same reason that properties linked with genes remain damaged when the genes have been damaged.

Furthermore, the connection of respiration with the grana (7) also explains carcinogenesis that I have not mentioned previously, the carcinogenesis is caused by x-rays. Rajewsky and Pauly have recently shown that the respiration linked with the grana can be destroyed with strong doses of x-rays, while the small part of the respiration that takes place in the fluid protoplasm can be inhibited very little by irradiation. Carcinogenesis by X-rays is obviously nothing else than destruction of respiration by elimination of the respiring grana.

It should also be mentioned here that grana, as Graffi has shown (8), fluoresce brightly if carcinogenic hydrocarbons are brought into their surroundings, because the grana accumulate the carcinogenic substances. Probably this accumulation is the explanation for the fact that carcinogenic hydrocarbons, although almost insoluble in water, can inhibit respiration and therefore have a carcinogenic effect.

When the respiration of body cells has been irreversibly damaged, cancer cells by no means immediately result. For cancer formation, there is necessary not only an irreversible dam aging of the respiration, but also an increase in the fermentation -- indeed, such an increase of the fermentation that the failure of respiration is compensated for energetically. But how does this increase of fermentation come about?

The most important fact in this field is that there is no physical or chemical agent with which the fermentation of cells in the body can be increased directly; for increasing fermentation, a long time and many cell divisions are al ways necessary. The temporal course of this increase of fermentation in carcinogenesis has been measured in many interesting works, among which I should like to make special mention of those of Dean Burk (9). Burk first cut out part of the liver of healthy rats and investigated the metabolism of the liver cells in the course of ensuing regeneration, in which, as is well known, the liver grows more rapidly than a rapidly growing tumor.

No increase of fermentation was found. Burk then fed rats for 200 days on yellow butter, whereupon liver carcinomas were produced, and he found that the fermentation slowly increased in the course of 200 days toward values characteristic of tumors.

The mysterious latency period of the production of cancer is, therefore, nothing more than the time in which the fermentation increases after a damaging of the respiration. This time differs in various animals: it is essentially long in man and here often amounts to several decades, as can be determined by the cases in which the time of the respiratory damage is known - for example, in arsenic cancer and irradiation cancer.

The driving force of the increase of fermentation, however, is the energy deficiency under which the cells operate after destruction of their respiration which forces the cells to replace the irretrievably lost respiration energy in some way. They are able to do this by a selective process that makes use of the fermentation of the normal body cells.

The more weakly fermenting body cells perish, but the more strongly fermenting ones remain alive, and this selective process continues until respiratory failure is compensated for energetically by the increase in fermentation. Only then has a cancer cell resulted from the normal body cell.

Now we understand why the increase in fermentation takes such a long time and why it is possible only with the help of many cell divisions. We also understand why the latency period is different in rats and in man. Since the average fermentation of normal rat cells is much greater than the average fermentation of normal human cells, the selective process begins at a higher fermentation level in the rat and, hence is completed more quickly than it is in man.

It follows from this that there would be no cancers if there were no fermentation of normal body cells, and hence we should like to know, naturally, from where the fermentation of the normal body cells stems and what its significance is in the body. Since, as Burk has shown, the fermentation remains almost zero in the regenerating liver growth, we must conclude that the fermentation of the body cells is greatest in the very earliest stages of embryonal development. Under these conditions, it is obvious - since ontogeny is the repetition of phylogeny-- that the fermentation of body cells is the inheritance of undifferentiated ancestors that have lived in the past at the expense of fermentation energy.

But why -- and this is our last question - are the body cells differentiated when their respiration energy is replaced by fermentation energy?

At first, one would think that it is immaterial to the cells whether they obtain their energy from respiration in or from fermentation, since the energy of both reactions is transformed into the energy of adenosine triphosphate, and yet adenosine triphosphate = adenosine triphosphate.

This equation is certainly correct chemically and energetically, but it is incorrect morphologically, because although respiration takes place for the most part in the structure of the grana, the fermentation enzymes are found for a great er part in the fluid protoplasm.

The adenosine triphosphate is synthesized by fermentation. Thus, it is as if one reduced the same amount of silver on a photographic plate by the same amount of light, but in one case with diffused light and in the other with patterned light.

In the first case, a diffuse blackening appears on the plate, but in the second case, a picture appears; however, the same thing happens chemically and energetically in both cases. Just as one type of light energy involves more structure than the other type, the adenosine triphosphate energy involves more structure when it is formed by respiration than it does when it is formed by fermentation.

In any event, it is one of the fundamental facts of present-day biochemistry that adenosine triphosphate can be synthesized in homogeneous solutions with crystallized fermentation enzymes, whereas so far no one has succeeded in synthesizing adenosine triphosphate in homogeneous solutions with dissolved respiratory enzymes, and the structure always goes with oxidative phosphorylation.

Moreover, it was known for a long time before the advent of crystallized fermentation enzymes and oxidative phosphorylation that fermentation -the energy supplying reaction of the lower organisms - is morphologically inferior to respiration. Not even yeast, which is one of the lowest forms of life, can maintain its structure permanently by fermentation alone; it degenerates to bizarre forms.

However, as Pasteur showed, it is rejuvenated in a wonderful manner, if it comes in contact with oxygen for a short time. "I should not be surprised," Pasteur said in 1886 (10) in the description of these experiments, "if there should arise in the mind of an attentive hearer a presentiment about the causes of those great mysteries of life which we conceal under the words youth and age of cells." Today, after 80 years, the explanation is as follows: the firmer connection of respiration with structure and the looser connection of fermentation with structure.

This, therefore, is the physiochemical explanation of the dedifferentiation of cancer cells. If the structure of yeast cannot be maintained by fermentation alone, one need not state that highly differentiated body cells lose their differentiation upon continuous replacement of their respiration with fermentation.

I would like at this point to draw attention to a consequence of practical importance. When one irradiates a tissue that contains cancer cells as well as normal cells, the respiration of the cancer cells, already too small, will decline further. If the respiration falls below a certain minimum that the cells need unconditionally, despite their increased fermentation, they die; whereas the normal cells, where respiration may be harmed by the same amount, will survive because, with a greater initial respiration, they will' still possess a higher residual respiration after irradiation. This explains the selective killing action of x-rays on cancer cells. But still further: the descendants of the surviving normal cells may in the course of the latent period compensate the respiration decrease by the fermentation increase and, thence, become cancer cells.

Thus it happens that radiation, which kills cancer cells, can also at the same time produce cancer, or that urethane, which kills cancer cells, can also at the same time produce cancer. Both events take place from harming respiration: the killing, by harming an already harmed respiration; the carcinogenesis, by the harming of a not yet harmed respiration

When differentiation of the body cells has occurred and cancer cells have there by developed, there appears a phenomenon to which our attention has been called by the special living conditions of ascites cancer cells. In extensively progressed ascites cancer cells of the mouse, the abdominal cavity contains so many cancer cells that the latter cannot utilize their full capacity to respire, and ferment because of the lack of oxygen and sugar. Nevertheless, the cancer cells remain alive in the abdominal cavity, as the result of transplantation proves.

Recently, we have confirmed this result by direct experiments in which we placed varying amounts of energy at the disposal of the ascites outside the body, in vitro, and then transplanted it. This investigation showed that all cancer cells were killed when no energy at all was supplied for 24 hours at 38 degrees Celsius but that one-fifth of the growth energy was sufficient to preserve the transplantability of the ascites.

This result can also be expressed by saying that cancer cells require much less energy to keep them alive than they do for growth. In this they resemble other lower cells, such as yeast cells, which remain alive for a long time in densely packed packets - almost without respiration and fermentation.

In any case, the ability of cancer cells to survive with little energy, if they are not growing, will be of great importance for the behavior of the cancer cells in the body.

Since the increase in fermentation in the development of cancer cells takes place gradually, there must be a transitional phase between normal body cells and fully formed cancer cells. Thus, for example, when fermentation has become so great that the respiration defect has been fully compensated for energetically by fermentation, we may have cells which indeed look like cancer cells but are still energetically insufficient. Such cells, which are clinically not cancer cells, have lately been found, not only in the prostate, but also in the lungs, kidney, and stomach of elderly persons. Such cells have been referred to as "sleeping cancer cells." (11, 12)

The sleeping cancer cells will possibly play a role in chemotherapy. From energy consideration, I could think that sleeping cancer cells could be killed more easily than growing cancer cells in the body, and that the most suitable test objects for finding effective agents would be the sleeping cells of the skin -that is, the precancerous skin.

Cancer cells originate from normal body cells in two phases. The first phase is the irreversible injuring of respiration. Just as there are many remote causes of plague --heat, insects, rats-- but only one common cause, the plague bacillus, there are a great many remote causes of cancer - tar, x-rays, arsenic, pressure, urethane - but there is only one common cause into which all other causes of cancer merge, the irreversible injuring of respiration.

The irreversible injuring of respiration is followed, as the second phase of cancer formation, by a long struggle for existence by the injured cells to maintain their structure, in which a part of the cells perish from lack of energy, while another part succeed in replacing the irretrievably lost respiration by fermentation energy. Because of the morphological inferiority of fermentation energy, the highly differentiated body cells are converted by this into undifferentiated cells that grow wildly - the cancer cells.

To the thousands of quantitative experiments on which these results are based, I should like to add, as a further argument, the fact that there is no alternative today. The explanation of a vital process is its reduction to physics and chemistry. There is today no other explanation for the origin of cancer cells, either special or general. From this point of view, mutation and carcinogenic agent are not alternatives, but empty words, unless metabolically specified. Even more harmful in the struggle against cancer can be the continual discovery of miscellaneous cancer agents and cancer viruses, which, by obscuring the underlying phenomena, may hinder necessary preventive measures and thereby become responsible for cancer cases.

The high fermentation of ascites cancer cells was discovered in Dahlem in 1951(12) and since then has been confirmed in many works (13,14). For best measurements, the ascites cells are not transferred to Ringer's solution but are maintained in their natural medium, ascites serum, which is adjusted physiologically at the beginning of the measurement by addition of glucose and bicarbonate. Because of the very large fermentation, it is necessary to dilute the ascites cells that are removed from the abdominal cavity rather considerably with ascites serum; otherwise the bicarbonate would be used up within a few minutes after addition to the glucose, and hence the fermentation would be brought to a standstill.

Under physiological conditions of pH and temperature, we find the following metabolic quotients in ascites serum (15):

$QQ(O_2)$	=	-5 to -10
$Q(M)(O_2)$	=	25 to 35
$Q(M)(N_2)$	=	50 to 70

where $Q(O_2)$ is the amount of oxygen in cubic millimeters that 1 milligram of tissues (dry weight) consumes per hour at 38 degrees Celsius with oxygen saturation, $Q(M)(O_2)$ is the amount of lactic acid in cubic millimeters that 1 milligram of tissue (dry weight) develops per hour at 38 degrees Celsius in the absence of oxygen. Even higher fermentation quotients have been found in the United States with other strains of mouse ascites cancer cells (13,14).

All calculations of the energy-production potential of cancer cells should now be based on quotients of the ascites cancer cells, since these quotients are 2 or 3 times as large anaerobically as the values formerly found for the purest solid tumors. The quotients of the normal body cells, however, remain as they were found in Dahlem in the years from 1924 to 1929 (16-19). It is clear that the difference in metabolism between normal cells and cancer cells is much greater than it formerly appeared to be on the basis of measurements of solid tumors.

Since the discovery of the oxidation reaction of fermentation in 1939 (20), we have known the chemical reactions by which adenosine diphosphate (A.D.P.) is phosphorylated to adenosine triphosphate in fermentation; and since then we have found that 1 mole of fermentation lactic acid produces 1 mole of adenosine triphosphate (A.T.P.).

The chemical reactions by which A.T.P. is synthesized in respiration are still unknown, but it can be assumed, according to the existing measurements (21), that 7 moles of A.T.P. can be formed when 1 mole of oxygen is consumed in respiration

A.T.P. quotients: If we multiply $Q(O_2)$ by 7 and $Q(M)(N_2)$ by 1, we obtain the number of cubic millimeters of A.T.P. that 1 milligram of tissue (dry substance) can synthesize per hour (22,400 cubic millimeters = 1 millimole of A.T.P.) We call these quotients

Q(A.T.P.) (O_2) and Q(A.T.P.)(N_2), according to whether the A.T.P. is formed by respiration or by fermentation, respectively.

Energy production of cancer cells and normal body cells: In Table 1, the Q values of some normal body cells are contrasted with the Q values of our ascites cancer cells.

The cancer cells have about as much energy available as the normal body cells, but the ratio of the fermentation energy to the respiration energy is much greater in the cancer cells than it is in the normal cells.

If a young rat embryo is transferred from the amniotic sac to Ringer's solution, the previously transparent embryo becomes opaque and soon appears coagulated (17). At the same time, the connection between respiration and phosphorylation is broken; that is, although oxygen is still consumed and carbon dioxide is still developed, the energy of this combustion process is lost for life. If the metabolism quotients had previously been in the amniotic fluid:

$$Q(O_2) = -15, Q(M)(O_2) = 25, Q(M)(N_2) = 25$$
$$Q(A.T.P.)(O_2) = 105, Q(A.T.P.)(N_2) = 25$$

afterward in Ringer's solution they are:

$$Q(O_2) = -15, Q(M)(O_2) = 25, Q(M)(N_2) = 25$$
$$Q(A.T.P.)(O_2) = 0, Q(A.T.P.)(N_2) = 25$$

Because of uncoupling of respiration and phosphorylation, the energy production of the embryo has fallen from Q(ZA.T.P.)(O_2) = Q(A.T.P.)(N_2) = 130, to 51; since the uncoupling is irreversible, the embryo dies in the Ringer's solution.

This example will show that the first phase of carcinogenesis, the irreversible damaging of respiration, need not be an actual decrease in the respiration quotient but merely an uncoupling of respiration, with undiminished overall oxygen consumption. Ascites cancer cells, which owe their origin primarily to an uncoupling of respiration, could conceivably have the following metabolism quotients, for example:

$$Q(O_2) = -50, Q(M)(O_2) = 100, Q(M)(N_2) = 100$$
$$Q(A.T.P.)(O_2), Q(A.T.P.)(N_2) = 100$$

which would mean that, despite great respiration, the usable energy production would be displaced completely toward the side of fermentation. One will now have to search for such cancer cells among the ascites cancer cells. Solid tumors - and especially solid spontaneous tumors- need no longer be subjected to such examinations today, of course, since the solid tumors are usually so impure histologically.

Aerobic fermentation is a property of all growing cancer cells, but aerobic fermentation (p.313) without growth is a property of damaged body cells - for example, embryos that have been transferred from amniotic fluid to Ringer's solution.

Since it is always easy to detect aerobic fermentation but generally difficult to detect growth, or lack thereof, of body cells, aerobic fermentation should not be used as a test for cancer cells, as I made clear in 1928 (19).

Nevertheless, misuse is still made of aerobic fermentation. Thus, O'Connor (22) recently repeated our old experiments on the aerobic fermentation of the embryo that has been transferred into Ringer's solution, but he drew the conclusion that the growth of normal body cells is completed at the expense of the aerobic fermentation, even though it has long been established that the embryo does not ferment aerobically when it grows in the amniotic fluid.

Short-period oxygen deficiency irreversibly destroys the respiration of embryos (1) without thereby inhibiting the anaerobic fermentation of the embryo. If such embryos are transplanted, teratomas are formed (31). It has recently been reported that, in the development of the Alpine salamander, malformations occurred when the respiration was inhibited by hydrocyanic acid in the early stages of embryonal development (32).

Goldblatt and Cameron (3) reported that, in the in vitro culturing of fibroblasts, tumor cells appeared when the cultures were exposed to intermittent oxygen deficiency for long periods, whereas, in the control cultures,no tumor cells appeared. In the discussion at the Stuttgart convention, Lettre cited against Goldblatt and Cameron the fact that another American tissue culturist, Earle, had occasionally obtained tumor cells from fibroblasts for reasons unknown to him and in an unreproduceable manner, but this objection does not seem weighty, and the latter part is un true (33). In any event, here is an area in which the methods of tissue culture could prove useful for cancer re search. But warnings must be given against metabolism measurements in tissue cultures, if and when the tissue cultures are mixtures of growing and dying cells, especially under conditions of malnutrition An example of the latter type of confusion is involved in the discussion by Al bert Fischer (34), especially in the chapter "Energy exchange of tissue cells cultivated in vitro."

Since this paper was prepared, striking confirmation and extension of its main conclusions have been obtained from correlated metabolic and growth studies of two lines of tissue culture cancer cells of widely differing malignancy that were both derived from one and the same normal, tissue culture cell (36). The single cell as isolated some 5 years ago from a 97- day old parent culture of a strain C_3H/ He mouse by Sanford, Likkely and Earle (33) of the National Cancer Institute.

Up to the time that the single-cell isolation was made, no tumors developed when cells of the parent culture were injected into strain C_3H/ He mice. Injections of in vitro cells of the lines 1742 and 049 (formerly labeled sub-strains VII and III, respectively) first produced tumors in normal C_3H/ He mice after the 12th and 19th in vitro transplant generations, respectively after 1.5 years, the percentage production of sarcomas was 63 and 0 percent, respectively, with correspondingly marked differences in length of induction period.

Despite such gross differences in "malignancy" in vivo, the rates of growth of the two lines of cells maintained continuously in vitro have remained nearly identical and relatively rapid. Nevertheless, the metabolism of the two lines of cancer cells, whose malignancy was developed in vitro, has been found by Woods, Hunter, Hobby, and Burk to parallel strikingly the differences in malignancy observed in vivo, in a manner in harmony with the predications and predictions of this article.

The metabolic values were measured following direct transfer of the liquid cultures from the growth flasks into manometric vessels, without notable alteration of environ mental temperature, pH, or medium composition (horse serum, chick embryo extract, glucose, bicarbonate, balanced saline). The values obtained this way accurately rep resent the metabolism of growing, adequately nourished, pure lines of healthy cancer cells free of admixture with any other tissue cell type. The anaerobic glycolysis of the high-malignancy line 1742 was $Q(M)N_2$ = 60 to 80, which is virtually maximum for any and all cancer cells previously reported, including ascites cells (12-14). The anaerobic glycolysis of the low-malignancy line was, however, only one-third as great, $Q(M)N_2$ = 20 to 30. The average aerobic glycolysis values for the two lines were in the the same order, $Q(M)O_2$ = 30 and 10, respectively, but of lower magnitude because of the usual, pronounced Pasteur effect, greater in line 1742 than in line 2049 ($Q(M)N_2 - Q(M)O_2$) = about 40 and 15). On the other hand, the rates of oxygen consumption were in converse order, being smaller in line 1742 ($Q(O_2)$ = 5 to 10) than in line 2049 ($Q(O_2)$ = 10 to 15), corresponding to a greater degree of respiratory defect in line 1742.

The respiratory defect in both lines was further delineated by the findings of little or no increase in respiration after the addition of succinate to either line of cells, in contrast to the considerable increases obtained with virtually all normal tissues (9); and the respiratory increase with paraphenylenediamine was likewise relatively low, compared with normal tissue responses.

A further notable difference between the two cell lines was the very much lower inhibition of glycolysis by podophyllin materials (anti-insulin potentiators) observed with line 1742 compared with line 2049 (for example, 10 and 70 percent, respectively, at a suitably low concentration). This result would be expected on the basis of the much greater loss of anti-insulin hormonal restraint of glucose metabolism, at the hexokinase phosphorylating level, as the degree of malignancy is increased, just as was reported for a spectrum of solid tumors (14).

Finally, the high-malignancy line 1742 cells have been found by A. L. Schade to contain 3 times as much aldolase as the low-malignancy line 2049 cells (11,300 versus 3700 Warburg activity units per millimeter of packed cells extracted), and about 2 times as much a-glycerophosphate dehydrogenase (600 versus 1400 Schade activity units (13) per millimeter of packed cells extracted). The potential significance of these indicated enzymic differences in relation to the parallel glycolytic differences, measured with aliquots of the same cell cultures, is evident, and may well be connected with the corresponding hexokinase system differences.

The new metabolic data on the two remarkably contrasting lines of cancer cells, which originated from a single, individual cell and have been maintained exclusively in vitro over a period of years, epitomize and prove finally the main conclusions of this article, which are based on decades of research. Such metabolic analyses provide promise of a powerful tool for diagnosis of malignancy in the ever-increasing variety of tissue culture lines now be coming available in this rapidly expanding biological and medical field, where characterization of malignancy by conventional methods (animal inoculation or otherwise) may be difficult or impracticable. This metabolic tool should be especially important in connection with the use of tissue cultures for the evaluation of chemotherapeutic agents or other control procedures.

REFERENCES AND NOTES

1. The transplantable ascites cancer was discovered by H. Loewenthal and G. Jahn (Z. Krebsforsch, 37,439 (1932)). G. Klein (Stockholm) expanded our knowledge about the physiology and morphology of the ascites tumors and showed their great advantages as experimental material. (Exptl. Cell Research, 2, 518 (1951))
2. F. Lynen, Naturwissenschaften 30, 398 (1942); Ann. 01.em. Justus Liebig 573, 60 (1951).
3. H. Goldblatt and G. Cameron, J. Exptl. Med, 97, 525 (1953).
4. O. Warburg, Pfluger's. Arch. Ges. Physiolo. 154,599 (1913); 158, 19 (1914).
5. C.D. Darlington, Brit. J. Cancer 2, 118 (1948).
6. M.W. Woods et al., J. Natl. Cancer Inst., 11, 1105 (1951); 9, 311 (19949); 9, 325 (1949); 16, 351 (1955). Science 102, 591 (1945); 111, 572 (1950). AAAS Research Conf. On Cancer (Science Press, Lancaster, Pa., 19945), p. 162. J. WASH. ACAD. SCI. 42, 169 (195). Pigment Cell Growth, M. Gordon, Ed. (Academic Press, New York, 1953), p.335. Biochem. Et Biophys. Acta 12, 329 (1953). Proc. Am. Ass. Cancer Research 1, 7 (1954). Proc. Soc. Exptl. Biol. Med. 83, 6 (1953). Phytopathology 33, 637, 766 (1943); 36, 47 (1946); 31, 978 (1941); 3, 288 (1942). Am. J. Botany 33, 12a (1946); 38, 419 (1951).
7. A compilation of American works on the grana, in which my results of 1914 (4) have been confirmed, is given by G. Hogeboom, W. Schneider, and M. Striebich in Cancer Research (133, 617 (1953)). In a very special case -- nucleated red blood cells of birds, which contain no grana or only poorly visible ones -the entire respiration can be cen-

trifuged off with the cell nuclei (O. Warburg, Hoppeseyler's Z. Physiol. Chem. 70, 413 (1913)).
8. A. Graffi, Z. Krebsforsch, 49, 477 (1939).
9. D. Burk, Symposium On Respiratory Enzymes (University of Wisconsin Press, Madison, 194), p.335. J. G. Kidd, R. J. Winzler, D. Burk, Cancer Research 4, 547 (1944).
10. L. Pasteur, Etudes Sur La Bierre (Masson, Paris, 1876), p. 240.
11. J. Craigie, J. Pathol. Bacteriol. 63, 177 (1951); 64, 251(1952). H. Hamperl, Verhandl. Deut. Ges. Pathol. 35, 9 (1951).
12. O. . Warburg And E. Hiepler, Z. Naturforsch 7b, 193 (1952).
13. Al. Shade, Biochim. Et. Biophys. Acta 12, 163 (1953).
14. M. Woods, J. Hunter, D. Burk, J. Natl. Cancer.
Inst. 16, 351(1955).
15. I am indebted to Georg Klein of the Karolinsska Institute, Stockholm Sweden, for his Ehrlich strain of mouse ascites cells.
16. O, Warburg, K. Posener, E. Negelein, Biochem. Z.
152, 309 (1924).
17. E. Negelein, Ibid, 165, 122 (1925).
18. O. Warburg et al., Ibid, 189, 114, 175, 242 (1924);
193, 315 (1928); 197, 175 (1928); 204, 475,479 (199).
19. O.Warburg, Ibid. 204, 482 (1929).
20. O. Warburg et al., Ibid. 303, 40, 132 (1939).
21. H.A. Krebs et al., Biochem. H. London 54, 107 (19953).
22. R.j. O'connor, Brit. J. Exptl.pathol. 31, 390 (1951).
23. O. Warburg, Hoppe-seyler's Z. Physiol. Chem. 70, 413 (1911); M. Onaka, Ibid. 70, 433 (1911); 71, 1933 (1911).
24. K. Dresel, Biochem. Z. 178, 70 (1926).
25. E. Negelein, Ibid. 165, 203 (1925).
26. D.N. Gupta, Nature 175, 257 (1955)..
27. R. Usui, Pfluger's Arch. Ges. Physiol. 147, 100 (1912).
28. O. Warburg, Hoppe-steyler's Z. Physiol. Chem. 66, 305 (1910); 70, 413 (1911).
29. ---,Biochem. 119, 143 (1921).
30. C.D. Larsen, J. Natl. cancer Inst. 8, 63 (1947). 31.
31. O. Warburg, Biochem. Z. 2288, 257 (1930).
32. H. Tiedemann And H. Tiedemann, Z. Naturs forsch. 9b, 371 (1954).
33. K. Sanford, G.d. Likely, W.R. Earle, J. Natl. Cancer Inst. 15, 15 (1954).
34. A. Fischer, Biology Of Tissue Culture (Copenhagen, Denmark, 1946).
35. O. Warburg, Biochem. Z. 160, 307 (1925); D. Burk et al., J. Natl. Cancer Inst. 2, 201 (1941).
36. This summary of studies of various collaborative groups of investigators was prepared by Dean Burk at Professor Warburg's request.

APPENDIX FOUR:
Uses for Stabilized Oxygen

> "New ideas pass through three periods: It can't be done. It probably can be done, but it's not worth doing. I knew it was a good idea all along !"
> Arthur C. Clarke.

Please Note: the following information is not intended to make any medical claims about the use of stabilized oxygen for any purposes. The testimonials that follow were unsolicited from consumers who have approached their health ailments and needs by using stabilized oxygen as a dietary supplement instead of, or in addition to, traditional medicines, over-the counter remedies or accepted surgical or medical procedures.

As one of the the largest sections in this book, these uses and testimonials are provided for the sole purpose of sharing what individuals are writing about stabilized oxygen supplementation. They represent a very small sampling of thousands of encouraging messages I have received over the last 25 years. For the most part, these testimonies are not supported by medical research, nor should you assume them as the recommendation of the use of any stabilized oxygen for any medical purposes or physiological issues.

All references, in the following testimonials, to specific brand name products, manufacturers or distributors have been replaced by the generic name "stabilized oxygen" to prevent the endorsement of any one brand or company over another.

Finally, please note that all of these individuals are referring to one specific category of stabilized oxygen supplementation, even though many different modalities were discussed in this book. Only the use of liquid dietary supplements that were pH balanced, and that contain levels of bioavailable oxygen in excess of 50,000 mg/L (p.p.m.), are listed on the following pages.

AGRICULTURAL OXYGEN APPLICATIONS

• Approximately 1 ounce of stabilized oxygen in one gallon of water can make an effective antimicrobial dip for fruits and vegetables. Stabilized oxygen acts as a topical disinfectant for surface disease organisms. Tests indicate a high destructive organism ratio - on contact - against most anaerobic molds, yeasts, fungi and bacteria.

• Flowers, foliage plants and ornamentals are susceptible to a variety of diseases like powdery mildew, black spot and rust. A 50% stabilized oxygen and 50% water solution, in a spray bottle, may help reduce, and in most cases eliminate, these problems. Reports of stabilized oxygen used on roses suffering from blights indicate a complete elimination of these problems in only two applications. The upper and lower surfaces of the foliage were sprayed in the early mornings or late evenings for best results. This spray is also effective on powdery mildew on snapdragons, beans, peas and strawberries.

• Add one gallon of stabilized oxygen to 30 gallons of water as a foliar feed. This mixture is sufficient to spray one acre of plants. Spray on plants early in the morning (4:00 to 8:00 a.m.) when the plant pores are open. Excellent results have been reported when used on soybeans, edible beans, corn, wheat and oats.

• Current plant research indicates that when oxygen rich water is added to a foliar feed spray on potatoes, this new solution enhances the plants' resistance to frost damage down to as low as minus 5° Celsius. Treating potatoes at five and one quarter quarts of stabilized oxygen in 20-30 gallons of water per acre resulted in a yield of six tons of potatoes per acre, mainly due to the fact that the treated potatoes continued to grow in spite of the frost, and that the untreated potatoes were frosted-off at the soil level.

• Diatomic oxygen and ozone are found in rain and snow and supply vital oxygen to all plant life. Research indicates that the oxidation process appears to stimulate protein production in growing plants. The benefits of higher oxygen concentrations in water supplies to vegetation include thicker plant stems and larger leaves. In standing crops, such as potatoes and corn, plant stems are thicker and stronger and the leaves are a brighter green color than those not receiving additional oxygen. Oxygen-nourished plants are believed to be more drought and disease resistant (especially to root-borne pathogens).

• All house plants can benefit from an increase in oxygenation. About seven teaspoons of stabilized oxygen added to two gallons of water will enhance the opening of flowers. Using 15 drops of stabilized oxygen in a vase of fresh cut flowers will keep the water fresher and clearer, will enhance flower appearance and life (up to 50% longer!), and will encourage flower opening. (Please note: soft tissue plants, such as tomatoes, should not be misted or sprayed with this mixture, as direct applications may result in scorch marks.)

• Spraying fruit trees at petal fall with full-strength stabilized oxygen may enhance fruit set. Subsequent sprays promote a higher growth rate, and the flavor of the treated fruit, when compared to untreated fruit from the same orchard, shows improvement in both quality and flavor.

• Some reports indicate that watering the ground around fruit trees with a solution of stabilized oxygen diluted in water may increase fruit yield. In some cases, trees that have not produced fruit for several seasons will bear fruit once again.

• To help germinate seeds, add eight ounces of stabilized oxygen to 16 ounces of distilled water. Soak the seeds for eight hours before planting. Some experiments with old wheat seeds resulted in an astonishing 90% germination rate compared to a control soaking in water that yielded only a 60% rate of germination.

• One gallon of stabilized oxygen in 1,000 gallons of water will increase the dissolved oxygen level the water to approximately 35 ppm (mg/L). This mixture ratio may be used for all farm animals including cattle, swine, poultry, sheep, goats, and rabbits. When used in this ratio for dairy cattle, results indicate an increase in milk production and butterfat content with reported less mastitis (an inflammation/infection of the udder) in the herds.

• Hog farmers report a shorter time preparing hogs for market, with an increased weight gain and less feed used. The drinking water is reported to be more clean and fresher, with a noticeable reduction in algae, bacteria and rust. There appears to be some control of the outbreak and spread of animal diseases as well.

- The use of stabilized oxygen in dairy farming was first recorded in 1985. At that time, stabilized oxygen was added to the polluted water system of one particular farm suffering from an outbreak of mastitis in the herd.

- One farmer recorded a significant reduction in the occurrence of mastitis as well as generally healthier cows. In 1988, one farmer stated that the butterfat content of his cows had in creased by 5.3%. Other farmers have reported production increases as high as eight pounds of butterfat per cow per milking, with bacteria counts as low as 2,000 per cubic centimeter.

- Stabilized oxygen can be used in the same way as a pipeline rinse for milk stone, depending on the length of the pipeline. As a rule, 14-24 ounces of stabilized oxygen should be added to 15 gallons of water, and used as a rinse. This ratio may also be used to rinse milk cans and the bulk milk tank to reduce bacteria levels.

- Stabilized oxygen may also be used as a completely safe and non-toxic udder wash in a ratio of eight ounces of stabilized oxygen to one gallon of warm water. Cows have soft, tender teats, and a dissolved oxygen-based formula of stabilized oxygen will not irritate the teat ends. The solution may be placed in a pump spray bottle and sprayed directly on the teats and the udder as often as needed to help reduce bacterial infection.

- Stabilized oxygen can be used as an additive to colostrum milk to reduce spoilage until it is to be used to feed newborn calves. Though the pH and temperature of the milk will vary, it is generally recommended that two ounces of stabilized oxygen be added per one gallon of colostrum milk.

- Newborn calves need extra oxygen. To facilitate this, add two ounces of stabilized oxygen to a bottle of calf milk twice a day (morning and evening). This appears to "brighten up" the calves, and in some cases reduces scours (diarrhea due to dysentery), which can lead to dehydration and/or death.

- Reports also indicate that stabilized oxygen, when added to the water of cows that have just calved, appears to "clean out", (i.e. helps to discharge out all of the placenta and afterbirth,) these cows much faster, thereby avoiding the infection which can result from retaining afterbirth material.

- An oxygen-rich drench can be used for cows with high fevers or for off-feed cows with mastitis. A solution of 14 ounces of stabilized oxygen to one quart of water has been used as a drench in the morning and in the evening over a three day period. In addition, stabilized oxygen may be applied directly to wounds on the skin surface to enhance the healing process.

- Stabilized oxygen has been used to convert crop residue into cattle feed. Residual crop items (straw, corn stalks, corn cobs, soybean residue, etc.) was treated with the direct application of stabilized oxygen. Mix one part of stabilized oxygen to 34 parts water and soak the residue material for 16 hours. This soaking process appears to breakdown fiber materials so that these residues may be more easily assimilated. Some feedlots have reported that the meat quality on animals fed using this process to be as good as those animals fed a diet of only corn.

- Slurry tanks are used by farmers to store animal wastes, usually wastes from dairy barns or hog operations. Odor is often a problem with these storage tanks. Research indicates that adding approximately 120 gallons of stabilized oxygen to every 350,000 gallons of slurry, and then agitating the slurry, will significantly reduce slurry odor. In some cases, the odor may even be completely eliminated.

- One gallon of stabilized oxygen may be added to one gallon of black strap molasses in 20 gallons of water per acre to use as a spray fertilizer enhancement to winter wheat crops for a higher and faster yield.

- Another farmer injected a solution of one gallon per acre of stabilized oxygen with 10 gallons of water with his corn seed at planting time. Even during a drought year, he harvested 130 bushels per acre, indicating that this mixture may have provided a measure of drought and stress protection to his crops..

- There is some research that indicates that treating herbicide-contaminated soils with a 50% solution of stabilized oxygen and water, over a two week period, may help neutralize these soil toxins. It is believed that the oxygen in this solution oxidizes the toxins and allows sensitive plants to grow in soil where previously they could not grow.

- Stabilized oxygen supplements are extremely potent and effective broad spectrum bactericide, fungicide, antiviral, and anti-parasitic compounds. They are environmentally safe with little or no toxicity to either man, fish, reptiles or animals.

- Stabilized oxygen may be used as a bactericide and fungicide in both pre-harvest and post-harvest treatment in aquacultural farming. Add 160 drops per gallon weekly for optimum bactericidal effect. Reports indicate that when added to water, the fungal growth rate in the tanks and on the fish is significantly reduced. A solution of approximately five to ten ppm of pH balanced stabilized oxygen will yield noticeable results. Tropical fish breeders have added one to two ounces of stabilized oxygen to 20 gallons of aquarium water to control microbial and algae growth.

- Stabilized oxygen is a mold inhibitor, is antibacterial, anti-fungal, antiviral and anti-parasitic. Wash aviary cages and feeder units with 50%-100% solution prior to each feeding.

- Stabilized oxygen can be used as an effective yet completely safe antimicrobial cage wash. Stabilized oxygen and sodium perborate were used by Robert Stroud (the famous "Bird Man of Alcatraz") to heal birds as reported in his book Diseases of Birds.

- Reports indicate that 10-20 drops of stabilized oxygen, added to hummingbird feeders, will reduce or eliminate fungal and bacterial growth around feeder tube openings. The addition of stabilized oxygen appears to act as a natural preservative, keeping the sugar solution fresher so that it will last longer.

- Stabilized oxygen may be used as a disinfectant for aquariums to minimize water contamination, as well as a water additive to inhibit microbial or algae build up. Add 80-160 drops of stabilized oxygen per one gallon of water.

- Research indicates that stabilized oxygen added to the drinking water of hogs results in meat that is more lean than the meat from hogs fed non-oxygenated drinking water. In some cases, hog fat content was lower than 10% of total body weight.

- Hogs are susceptible to various diseases, including pneumonia. These diseases are held in check with the use of various antibiotics. Stabilized oxygen appears to reduce the need to use large doses of antibiotics. Also, hogs that drink water treated with stabilized oxygen are reported to have healthier respiratory systems and are subject to fewer diseases. Hogs with scours (diarrhea due to dysentery) have been treated with a solution of approximately one half ounce of stabilized oxygen per gallon of drinking water for three days. Then the mixture was reduced to approximately 15 ounces of stabilized oxygen per gallon of water for daily maintenance.

- Tests indicate that stabilized oxygen added to poultry drinking water may reduce the outbreak and severity of the avian flu virus. In addition, stabilized oxygen has been reported to increase egg production in those hens drinking treated water with a higher oxygen content. Some poultry farmers have reported that chickens drinking treated water have reduced occurrences of breast blisters and the heavier chickens experienced a significant reduction in tendon breakage.

- One turkey farm in Canada reported that its birds had a lower mortality rate, consumed 8 1/2% less feed, yet averaged 1 1/2 pounds more weight per bird because of the use of oxygen treated drinking water.

- Washing boiler carcasses in stabilized oxygen has been shown to reduce the levels of salmonella contamination. One study, reported in Poultry Science (Issue 66, 1987) resulted in a noticeable reduction in salmonella after a ten minute dip in a 1% solution of stabilized oxygen.

- In another test, broiler carcasses were soaked for ten minutes in a 50% solution of stabilized oxygen and water. Tests indicate that the salmonella bacteria levels were reduced and in some cases completely eliminated.

- Stabilized oxygen may be used as an antimicrobial disinfectant wash for reptiles, reptile cages and as a hand wash for pre- and post handling. Use from full strength to 50% strength. A pump spray bottle was be used for dispersion.

- Stabilized oxygen may also be used as a mold inhibitor, as well as an antibacterial, anti-fungal, antiviral, and anti-parasitic wash for feeder units. Feeder units and tanks were washed with a 50%-100% solution prior to each feeding or filling as a natural, yet safe, disinfectant.

- Stabilized oxygen reduced the incidence of Alternaria zinniae on zinnia seeds. Control seeds (0%) had 85% (17 of 20) while seeds soaked for 48 hours in a 100% solution of stabilized oxygen had 20% (4 of 20) with A. zinniae. Conidia or hyphae contaminating the surface of the zinnia seeds were probably killed by the stabilized oxygen, but hyphae within the seed coat probably escaped. Germination rates tended to be increased by the stabilized oxygen, although our results did not show an increased germination rate with soaking for 48 hours in a 100% solution of stabilized oxygen. Control seeds soaked for 48 hours had a 65% (13 of 20) germination while seeds soaking for 24 hours in stabilized oxygen had a 90% (18 of 20) germination. Under conditions where seed lots are heavily infested with Alternaria zinniae, seed disinfection with stabilized oxygen prior to seeding can reduce the incidence of damping off and blight of zinnia.

• Additionally, seed germination rates would be increased, resulting in many more healthy plants. With the additional characteristics of having no toxicity to humans or animals and being biodegradable, stabilized oxygen Activated oxygen shows promise being used as a disinfectant of fruits and vegetables and other food products in addition to being used to produce clean seeds and increase seed germination rates.

• Dr. M. Yoshimura , Ph. D. , School of Biological Sciences, Phytopathology Department, California Polytechnic State University, San Luis Obispo, CA U.S.A.

• It was noted that the wholesale buyers of the chickens were very impressed with the flavor of the stabilized oxygen treated chickens in this study. The reasons, the Doctors believe, is that the oxygen from stabilized oxygen helps build stronger immune systems and therefore bacteria and parasites are controlled to a higher degree. The treated chickens are more active and thereby develop more as well as stronger muscles resulting in less fat. The improved quality of the meat and the lack of Antibiotics used as a result of stabilized oxygen treatment might allow the producer to market the chickens as "Organic" thereby reaching higher sales prices and more demand. Overall, this has been a very successful preliminary study and points towards areas that need to be examined further. The positive results of increased growth, weights, less mortality, overall improved health and vitality of the chickens, improved flavor of the meat in taste tests and improved acceptability of the end products were all observed in this study. Another parallel stabilized oxygen study was conducted with exotic birds that also indicates an increased health benefit across the board and increased survivability of hatching eggs.
Dr. A. Rotou, DVM

• Aphenomyces is a fungus that has been attacking sugar beet (Beta vulagris) fields in the Red River Valley of Minnesota and North Dakota. The organism is soil borne and may affect the sugar beets from the early season seedling stage until the late summer more mature stage. This study shows the effect of stabilized oxygen on aphenomyces in petri dish cultures and soil. From the above tables. one can see that stabilized oxygen at all concentrations had an adverse effect on Aphenomyces growing in petri dish cultures. It can also be seen that at the highest concentration most of the Aphenomyces were killed.
Dr. C. Habstritt, Ph.D., Professor of Agronomy & Soils, University of Minnesota

- Rusty, our huge and magnificent tabby, came to us, like all our pets, as an orphan in need. He was about two years old and accustomed to fending for himself. We healed a large abscess under his chin by cleansing and spraying the area with a two percent solution of stabilized oxygen. We treated his snake-bitten paw, swollen to triple size, with the same solution. Both heatings were complete within two to three days, as was a deep cut between his eyes.
E.S., AZ U.S.A.

- I have two little four-legged critters, cockapoos. One is nearly 14, and the other is almost eight years old. I apportioned them a dosage of stabilized oxygen, based on their weights relative to mine, and I'm glad to say that the older one is much more peppy, her breath is sweeter, and the tongue of each of them is distinctly pinker (as in more oxygen in their circulatory system.) Since I don't know the color of my tongue before I started taking stabilized oxygen, I can make no comparison!! My vet recently saw the older of the dogs and could hardly believe that she was the age that she is. She runs all over the place, jumps up on the sofa, and goes right over the arm at the end, down to the floor, and repeats a loop around the living room. She's like the Energizer Bunny! So, you can be sure that I will continue to take stabilized oxygen and give it to my dogs...
J.S., CA U.S.A.

ATHLETIC PERFORMANCE: OXYGEN STAMINA, ENDURANCE, ENERGY, RECOVERY

- Whether you are a world-class athlete or a recreational runner, your capacity for endurance exercise has similar physiological limitations. Endurance exercise can be defined as the ability to perform cardiovascular exercise, whether it be cross-country skiing, spinning, running, aerobic exercise or swimming, for an extended period of time..Despite the multifaceted nature, endurance exercise is characterized by one simple requirement – the necessity to sustain repeated muscle contraction. This

criterion is fulfilled through two basic functions – the ability to consume enough oxygen and an adequate fuel provision.[197]
Dr. Len Kravitz, Ph.D

• A first principle in exercise physiology is that work requires energy, and to maintain a specific work rate or running velocity over a long distance, ATP must be supplied to the cross bridges as fast as it is used. As the duration of an all-out performance increases there is greater reliance on ATP production via oxidative phosphorylation to maintain cross bridge cycling. Consequently, the rate at which oxygen is used during prolonged submaximal exercise is a measure of the rate at which ATP is generated.[198]
Dr. Bassett, Ph.D. & Dr. Howley, Ph.D.

• I have noticed an improved performance at track training since I've been taking stabilized oxygen. I was really pushing it and my legs were screaming with the efforts but I was still able to maintain the cadence and repeat the efforts after a rest period. Recovery and well-being is noticeable using stabilized oxygen. I have been able to sleep better after late night training and I feel more relaxed and happy. After taking stabilized oxygen for nearly three weeks I can report that across the board the benefits have been that I can operate at 6-8 beats HR higher, feel much more relaxed, able to sleep better & feel more invigorated. I am not experiencing the energy spikes/mood problems when hard training.
J. Austin, World Cycling Record Holder, Australia

• After months of vigorous training and preparation, our team set out to conquer Mt. Everest this past April and May (2013). Unless you actually see the breathtaking beauty of the Himalayas yourself, you have no concept of their awesomeness, beauty as well as their danger. Towering more than 29,000 feet (8,848 meters) into the sky, Mt. Everest has challenged the best-of-the-best for sixty years since Sir Edmund Hillary and Tenzing Norgay made history back in 1953. But above 24,600 feet (7,500 meters) is what we climbers call the 'death zone' where the oxygen level is insufficient to sustain life. Without supplemental oxygen, any climber would perish quickly. Of the more than 200 recorded deaths on the mountain, most were due to oxygen deprivation and exhaustion. Preparing for this exhilarating

---

[197] The Physiological Factors Limiting Endurance Exercise Capacity (MORE)
http://www.unm.edu/~lkravitz/Article%20folder/limitations.html

[198] Limiting factors for maximum oxygen uptake and determinants of endurance performance. Medical Science Sports Exercise (MORE)
http://www.ncbi.nlm.nih.gov/pubmed/10647532

and dangerous expedition meant that I had to develop techniques to improve my oxygen efficiency and reduce the effects of exhaustion. I turned to stabilized oxygen as a nutritional source to supplement my oxygen intake and took it multiple times every day. The results were beyond my expectations. I know that this supplement helped to make the difference in achieving my goal to stand at the top of the world. I could not have done it without stabilized oxygen as part of my survival gear.
I. Gissurarson, World Class Mountain Climber, Iceland

• I have been using stabilized oxygen for only a short time and find it unreal.
B. Alders, National Rodeo Champion

• Since using stabilized oxygen I have been able to take my training to the next level, translating into improved results.
C. Winn - Team Yeti, Champion Cyclist, Australia

• Having researched the benefits of oxygen, I tried stabilized oxygen and was amazed at the difference it made to my energy, endurance and alertness at training. It's a winner.
A. Watt, Four Time World Kickboxing Champion

• My duet partner and myself recently discovered stabilized oxygen and were immediately intrigued …considering our sports, Synchronized Swimming, relies heavily on available oxygen. We first tried stabilized oxygen during competition, and were amazed by the results. We both agreed that it boosted our performance dramatically, especially towards the end of the program when fatigue really takes its toll. We felt as though we could continue to push ourselves harder throughout the whole routine, without "hitting the wall" at the end. Thank you for making available such a wonderful product, we now feel we are well on our way to begin the Australian duet to compete at the Beijing Olympics 2008.
E. Amberger and S. Bombell, Olympic Synchronized Swimmers

• From the results it is concluded that the ingestion of the stabilized oxygen solution considerably affects the tolerance levels of lactate acid in the blood and improves VO2max.
N. Pericleous, Trainer, M.Sc., ACSM

• I am a marathon runner. My PR is a 3:08:0 at the 1993 St. George Marathon. Prior to that time, my PR was a 3:16:20 (also at the St. George Marathon). I attribute this improvement to the use of stabilized oxygen. My training, weight, and all other factors were very similar as I checked my

training logs. I have to attribute the eight minute improvement to stabilized oxygen. I just felt better!
J.D.B., UT U.S.A.

- I have been involved in professional sports for the last 17 years, both at a professional level and a performance coaching level. Stabilized oxygen is probably the biggest breakthrough I've seen in those 17 years. Take control... Take stabilized oxygen.
T. Brigstock, PGA Golf Pro

- The potential role of stabilized oxygen stabilized liquid oxygen as an ergogenic aid in sports performance enhancement is still to be fully understood. Available scientific data and information on this subject presents a whole range of possibilities fur further studies. In this study it was established that...a definite improvement was noticed between the sprints of the trials with placebo and the controlled stabilized oxygen stabilized liquid oxygen. This would indicate the fact that athletes who consumed stabilized oxygen stabilized liquid oxygen were able to reproduce similar and sustained effort during both sprints as compared to those that consumed the placebo.
Dr. H. Zaheer, Ph.D., Sports Medicine & Research Centre, Department of Youth & Sports, Brunei Darussalam

- With regular stabilized oxygen use and increased dosage immediately before a race, I have noticed in creased endurance, strength and aerobic capacity. I look forward to my first long course competition in the San Luis Wildflower Triathlon next May.
LS., CA U.S.A., nationally ranked triathlete

- I believe stabilized oxygen, because of its inherent "energy factor" potential may just be the "Rosetta Stone" that unblocks the pathogenetic mechanisms of disease in general and provides the knowledge for proper disease prevention management. Stabilized oxygen is not simply an important nutrient supplement but a dynamic energy molecule. Stabilized oxygen has an extremely high ORP (Oxidation Reduction Potential) of 950 mV. That means stabilized oxygen possesses energy that can be transferred to the surrounding environment, potentiating the bioenergetic processes and correcting or reversing underlying cellular dysfunctions. In other words, stabilized oxygen works like a bright new cellular battery.
Dr. M. Spartalis, M.D., Vascular Surgeon

- Stabilized oxygen is undoubtedly a new powerful tool in the modern world of medicine. The more we get to know about it, the more we can

treat without side effects. Stabilized oxygen is a tool, a key to a noble dream for a better world, better life quality and life itself.
Dr. M. Christofinis, M.D., Ph.D., Academy of Medical Sciences, Berlin, Germany

- Since using stabilized oxygen I have found a number of benefits from the supplementation. The benefiting factor that I have noticed was increased long lasting energy.
B. Livermore, Olympic Hockey, Australia

- Stabilized oxygen contributed to me feeling energetic in the water. Glad to have found such a helpful, natural and drug-free product.
G. Workman, Triathlon Champion

- I used stabilized oxygen at the recent Australian Masters Track and Road Championship and won 3 gold and 3 silver medals.
K. Oliver, 6-Time World Masters Champion

- Without a doubt, I have seen an increased level of stamina and energy during my workouts and a reduction in recovery time post workout. I have…rigorously used stabilized oxygen personally, coming to the conclusion that this product is of the highest efficacy and has improved my physical performance.
S. Payton, NFL Head Coach, New Orleans' Saints

- I use stabilized oxygen everyday of my life. I feel it improves my game on the ice and I don't feel winded or tired. Especially in the third period.
R. Kesler, Forward, Vancouver Canucks, Olympic Silver Medalist, Team USA

- The Pepperdine Women's basketball program has been fortunate enough to utilize stabilized oxygen water during our season. We have used it in our pregame hydration program, and during the competition. The student athletes have all stated that they had a sharper mental edge, and a sustained physical stamina during their competitions. The results from using stabilized oxygen have met and exceeded our expectations, and this is not just your ordinary water. Stabilized oxygen (water) hydrates quickly and seems to really clear the mind for our games. I even see a major difference in my focus as a coach in my decision making process during the heat of games when using stabilized oxygen for pregame and during the game. As a program we see the difference between sports drinks and stabilized oxygen (water) and we will continue to use it in the future.
R. Weisenberg, Head Coach Women's Basketball, Pepperdine University

- I am a big cycling enthusiast and triathlete which helps me perform at my max when I sit in a race car...A few weeks ago I received a box of stabilized oxygen to test...it is safe to say the difference was noted immediately...I not only broke my personal record, but was in the top 20 of 4,950 people in my four mile interval, which topped at 33 mph. Everyone in my triathlon team has been asking what my secret is and I just giggle and say "water and air" and wink...This is the next big thing in performance sports worldwide.

Gustavo Menezes, Formula 3 Champion

- I am of the "no pain, no gain", workout regime. I have been looking for something for years that would take the pain away. I have found it! Stabilized oxygen water is bottled water with an oxygen supplement that really works for me. It makes my ankles, knees, arms shoulders, and hips recover more quickly than anything else I have ever tried. Every player I work out with, loves it because it is natural, tastes good and makes them feel better. I have shared it with many pro athletes and they are never without it now. I highly recommend stabilized oxygen.

Jim Harrick. Head Basketball Coach – University of Georgia. Former UCLA Coach, NCAA Champion 1995

- B.J. Lee is a national Hero in South Korea. He has won the Boston Marathon, was a silver medalist in the Atlanta Olympic Games and has been a top medalist in Asian Pacific and African competitions. Lee was voted the No. 1 marathon runner in the world by Track & Field News. He's now a huge fan of our stabilized oxygen brand in South Korea.

Lee Bong-Ju
Olympic Marathon Medalist

PHYSIOLOGY & DERMATOLOGY

- Thank you for giving me the honor here today to address during this seminar my experiences of using stabiliZed oxygen in dermatology. Oxygen was and remains the most basic element of all life forms we know, throughout centuries. Combined with hydrogen, it forms water; another precious source of life due to oxygen. The human body consists of 70% water in which oxygen has to have a concentration in order to maintain good health and skin conditions.

Water has been getting worse and worse during the last fifty years, affecting directly its quality and the concentration in oxygen min water. So, new forms of oxygen supply are needed now more than ever before.

But at the same time, I believe, that it is going to be even more true in the future.

The ancient Greeks described thousands of years ago the three most precious elements for all life-forms: Air, water and fire. Today we realize this truth, and attempt to solve the puzzle of these components. By saying "Air", the Greeks meant oxygen, of course. By "Water", again they referred to the power of oxygen. "Fire" cannot exist without oxygen necessary for the burning process. The ancient "coded message" to search and find a "stronger oxygen". The search for this long lasting oxygen has taken centuries.

So today, we have "stabilized oxygen" which was released in 1986. Thanks to a dedicated group of "sleepless and courageous scientists" in the USA, we have stabilized oxygen. The main achievement is an oxygen-rich solution that is stabilized and energized! It is FDA approved and it has been proven to exists and work.

What is actually "activated stabilized oxygen"? It is a rich source of bio-available free oxygen in a saline based solution. Current research studies indicate that it enhances metabolic energy, alertness and endurance. Some of the energy is used to generate (ATP) Adenosine Triphosphate, the main energy source for all muscle contractions, as well as cellular metabolic activities are derived from the breakdown of pyruvic acid. This decomposition process, occurs only in the presence of sufficient amounts of oxygen. ATP and oxygen react with pyruvic acid to become carbon dioxide and water.

So, "stabilized oxygen" is the safest, purest way to transport energy in cells, complexes and organs all over the human body.

Where can we use stabilized oxygen in dermatology? It is a very big subject, but I'll speak about my own experiences during the last 3 years in Cyprus.

We have had very good results healing open wounds (ulcera crurum), because of the improvement in the micro- and macro-circulation in the blood vessels using both topical and oral application of stabilized oxygen drops. At the same time, stabilized oxygen works as a strong antiseptic on the wound killing anaerobic organisms including fungals. Stabilized oxygen increases the healing process.

We have had excellent results using dilutions and for the oral treatment of Stomatitis Aphthosa in the mouth and gums. We have used stabilized oxygen in topical treatments against oral Candidiasis and tongue fungal plaques. We have seen dramatic improvements on degenerative lip dermatitis and Angulus Infectiosus in mouth angles.

Using stabilized oxygen on chronic Vaginitis Cardidomycetica, we believe that we have really made a major step forward and helped a number of very desperate women suffering from this common disease. We have used a stabilized oxygen solution enriched with liposomes, treating one woman only three times weekly in cycles of two weeks and obtaining remarkable results.

To treat psoriasis vulgaris focuses, we used creams containing stabilized oxygen plus liposomes for topical treatments. This formula was applied twice daily on areas without scabs so the absorption with the liposomes could reach the deeper layers of the dermis. We had satisfactory and very good results even complete remission.

On nail structural keratin problems, we used stabilized oxygen with liposomes and biotin and had remarkable results on Onycholysis, Onycholisis Semilunaris, and quicker nail growth.

Stabilized oxygen is undoubtedly a new powerful tool in the modern world of medicine. The more we get to know about it, the more beneficial we can treat without side effects. It is a tool, a key to a noble dream for a better world, better life quality and life itself.
Dr. M. L. Christofinis, M.D., Ph.D., Specialist Dermatologist & V.D., Academy of Sciences of Berlin, Member of German Society of Dermatology, Andrology & Phlebology

- In the beginning I used stab oxygen rather cautiously for cleaning the face for local uses thus assessing the action of this product as a bactericide. Later I started recommending it for the detoxification of the organism thus testing its activity for neutralizing free radicals. I gave it to my patients with tired and rather lifeless skin, with black circles under the eyes or individuals suffering from eczema and dermatitis. The results were fantastic and this made me bolder and able to recommend it to athletes, smokers, persons with feebleness, lack of energy, chronic bronchitis, asthma and to people with frequent viral infections due to a weakness in their immune system as well as to patients with bed-sores, etc. In all these cases the results have been excellent.
Dr. M. Chilindri, M.D., Pathology and Dermatology

- From my clinical experience this product can be used in all aspects of the oral medicine and surgery, for example: as an irrigant for the cleaning and prophylaxis of the oral cavity; for the treatment of periodontitis and gingivitis; for post surgical procedures and post extracting treatment; for biological treatment and elimination of amalgam filling and heavy metal drainage; for therapy in a systemic disease, and many other applications. In conclusion, I would like to say that stabilized oxygen, because of its biofriendly capabilities, has the potential to be a powerful source for clinical or paramedical practice.
Dr. S. Panayiotis, M.D.

CONSUMERS SPEAK OUT

• I wanted to thank you for introducing me to stabilized oxygen. I have been taking it for over six years and I would not be without it. I have trouble with bad gums and I keep that problem in tact with the oxygen and I take it when I have a cold, sore throat and to stave off all sorts of health problems. I think it is a wonder drug. I also use it for cuts, scratches and burns, even sunburns.
B. Shannon, Sarasota Fl.

• I bought your stabilized oxygen product for my mother from your distributor in Medellin, Colombia. She is 86 and the results have been great.
J. Maya, Quito, Ecuador

• My grandfather feels really great after taking this water. He is increasing the amount of mix to the water!
J. Kim, USA

• By using stabilized oxygen, my whole family is energetic. It boosts our immune systems. Thank you GOD for having this kind of OXYGEN SUPPLEMENT.
A. Darunday, Phillipines

• My mother is 80 years young and cant go a day without her liquid stabilized oxygen. Thank you!
J. Hamre, Hillsboro, ND

• I have been a medical researcher, both of Allopathic (Western) and Complimentary (Alternative) and Energy Medicine for over 35 years and have worked with Holistic doctors in a clinic setting. The theory of oxygenation of the blood, the body, as treatment for pathogens (which are mainly anaerobic) has great validity and been well proven. The difficulty to date has been the refusal of north american main stream medicine to acknowledge these results. Also for the ordinary person to self administer this type of therapy when in ill health has been difficult. Your new product is a god send and I will be disseminating the information about this product as widely as possible. I have worked to help others to create health in their bodies through life style, and food choices, and support the organic movement. Thank you for producing a product that will allow those who wish to be responsible in creating health from illness in their own body now have a method that is simple and affordable. Especially for cancer, which is increasing in North America.
J. Redden, U.S.A.

- I put about 40 drops of stabilized oxygen in a 20 oz. bottle and you can feel the difference, I even got one for my mother who smokes and she now breathes better. Love it.
D. Marie, North Carolina, USA

- 5 out of 5 stars. Because water will likely be the most important thing that you will ever store, making sure your water storage solution won't compromise the water is paramount! Forget bleach! It leaves a taste and can affect the container you store the water in. Unlike bleach, stabilized oxygen doesn't taste anything and won't affect the container.
B. LeRoy, San Francisco, CA U.S.A.

- I got this for my friend who has stage four cancer. She swears it helps keep her energy level up.
K. Daughtry, U.S.A.

- Best stuff to use and is tasteless for storing water. From 5 to 7 years.
M. Wilson, U.S.A.

- I wanted to thank you for introducing me to stabilized oxygen. I have been taking it for over six years and I would not be without it. I have trouble with bad gums and I keep that problem in tact with the oxygen and I take it when I have a cold, sore throat and to stave off all sorts of health problems. I think it is a wonder drug. I also use it for cuts, scratches and burns, even sunburns.
B. Shannon, Sarasota, Fl

- My mother is 80 years young and cant go a day without her liquid oxygen.
J. Hamre, Hillsboro, ND U.S.A.

- I have been on antibiotics off and on my whole life and I have suffered from Candida. The only way I am able to keep it in control is with stabilized oxygen. I now have more energy and less fatigue.
B.S., UT U.S.A.

- I was diagnosed with the Epstein-Barr virus and suffered from tremendous headaches and serious fatigue. After going to a regular M.D., I finally received my first dose of stabilized oxygen from a homeopathic specialist. The headaches began to subside and the fatigue gradually improved ...The stabilized oxygen now gives me more energy and my whole body feels much less fatigued.
S.K., UT U.S.A.

- I have absolutely no hesitation in recommending stabilized oxygen to my patients as an integral part of their overall therapies to rebuild their immune systems and metabolic processes. It has proved to be completely safe and I have had no incidents of com plications. I highly recommend stabilized oxygen as a daily supplement for everyone, not just those who have health problems.
K.H., D.C., D.I.C.A.K., UT U.S.A.

- I have suffered with poison oak every time I ride out in the mountains. I rubbed a stabilized oxygen solution of about one quarter stabilized oxygen with three-quarters water, and overnight, the poison oak was gone!
D.M., CA U.S.A.

- Last year my son sent me a bottle of stabilized oxygen and I started taking the product immediately. Over a four month period I gradually increased my dosage from seven drops to 55-60 drops a day. I can now work outdoors four to six hours a day without an asthma attack. I seldom, if ever, use my atomizer and I think stabilized oxygen has also increased my levels of energy, alertness, and has improved my memory.
T.O., OR U.S.A.

- Hot grease that splashed on my hand-I used stabilized oxygen on it with cotton balls until it quit hurting in approximately 15 minutes. All the pain was gone and there was NO SCAR!
R.E., UT U.S.A.

- Last week I was in agony when a patch of psoriasis (covering the entire instep and ankle of my left foot,) became infected, swollen and bleeding. This happened in spite of using every ointment, herbal tea remedy imaginable. I prepared a two percent solution of stabilized oxygen and immersed the entire foot for 25 minutes. All night I continued to feel pain. But by morning a great change had taken place! No swelling!
M.P., CA U.S.A.

- I have a severe chronic inflammatory condition that began in my late twenties. This condition has caused severe headaches, chronic fatigue, digestive problems and at times I am barely able to move, although I am not chronologically old…I have tried many alternative remedies but until taking stabilized oxygen had not seen such immediate positive results. I have been taking stabilized oxygen for 10 days. Prior to this I was having a severe flare up, but due to complications had been told to avoid medications. Ten days may not seem like a long time for a test, but for me a week without pain is like a miracle. I am not exhausted all the time and have more energy. It has been great to be pill free.

M.E., CA U.S.A.

• My mother suffers from migraine headaches and has been taking stabilized oxygen for several months. During this time the headaches have stopped. When she ran out of stabilized oxygen for several days, the head aches started up again. Needless to say, she takes stabilized oxygen on a regular basis.
F.J., CA U.S.A.

• For 14 years, I have battled "Athlete's Foot", and, in spite the best of the over-the-counter remedies, such as Lotrimin, and the much stronger prescription salves, I was always on the losing side of the battle. Even after following all directions (multiple applications/day for 2-3 weeks), the fungus always came back in the form of red, itchy spaces between my toes, and, much of the time, the red/ itchy areas only diminished and never really disappeared. I decided to try stabilized oxygen. I began with lightly rubbing 5-6 drops into each of the "infected" areas, once in the morning, and again at bedtime. In just 3 days I noticed improvement, and decided to continue the same treatment regimen. Within eight days, I neither saw nor felt the Athlete's foot. No more itchy feet! Now to keep the fungus at bay, I apply the stabilized oxygen drops only once a day, and I have yet to see in 9 weeks any more of that irritating problem. WHAT A RELIEF!
J.R., NV U.S.A.

• I have eczema on my hands. I have tried other products, but nothing has worked. The stabilized oxygen has given me relief. As soon as the eczema starts to flare up, I use the stabilized oxygen and the itch and rash never materialize.
P.L., CA U.S.A.

• Besides stabilized oxygen being used as an internal bactericide, viricide, and fungicide, it can be used topically for burns and rashes. Also it can aid in combat ing parasites ...It can be used to improve almost all health problems .
Dr. C.L., Ph.D., N.D., UT U.S.A.

• Stabilized oxygen has increased my alertness and energy levels. Smoking took my breath away and stabilized oxygen gave it back.
E.N., CA U.S.A.

• Last week, while cleaning my garage, I picked up an empty milk carton and felt a sudden sting on my hand. When I turned the carton upside-down, a small black spider tumbled out, and I stepped on it promptly. I assume it was a black widow spider, very common in this area. I hurried

into the house and applied stabilized oxygen concentrate directly on the bite area. Within five minutes the pain was gone and the red streak up my arm was no longer visible.
V.R., AZ U.S.A.

- I suffer with a rather rare variety of lung disease which has severely impaired my right lung. Stabilized oxygen seems to help so far.
W.B., SD U.S.A.

- Late in the day last Tuesday I noticed that my son Adam, five years old, had a few bumps on his face and chest. We had been sitting on the lawn so I assumed they were bug bites. The next morning he woke up with a raging case of chicken pox. He looked as though he had been boiled; bright red from his chin down to his feet, his feet so swollen that he could hardly walk, oozing pustules on his thighs, arms, chest and buttocks, dark red welts where ever his skin creased. He was tormented with itching and cried off and on for hours, complaining that he was on fire. At mid-morning I put him in a tepid bath, tub fairly full, with about two cups of stabilized oxygen added. This helped somewhat....When I spoke with the nurse at the doctor's office I was told that chicken pox runs about seven days. The next morning, Thursday, Adam bounced into our room at the crack of dawn singing and dancing...and feeling his usual self. All of the redness was gone and the only indication that he had had chicken pox were the dried and healing pustules. By Friday, these too were gone.
S.S., OR U.S.A.

- My sinuses, which have been infected since about 1940, are under control. They still discharge pus, especially now in the hay fever season, but it no longer makes me ill. My asthma, which dates back to the same period, is almost totally gone.
Rev. P.D., CA U.S.A.

- I can't thank you enough for introducing me to stabilized oxygen. This miraculous product has definitely improved my sense of well-being. I feel more energized, less nervous and feel confident that stabilized oxygen has reduced the harmful toxins in my body. I have applied it directly to my skin to relieve the pain caused by burns and bites, and I feel that I have lost weight as a result in taking your product. I can never thank you enough.
G.T., CA U.S.A.

- I can tell you that stabilized oxygen has eliminated a painful plantar wart from the ball of my left foot thereby obviating laser surgery. I am delighted!

B.R., CA U.S.A.

- I wish to express my gratitude for your product. It seems my heart wasn't getting enough oxygen and after consulting my doctor I gave stabilized oxygen a try. It, plus the herb hawthorne, saved me from taking digitalis for the rest of my life. I am 75 years old and feel young again. I wish everybody could have some of this wonderful stabilized oxygen!
V.J., CA U.S.A.

- During the past year, I have had several bladder infections, sometimes reoccurring after two weeks. Previously, I had gone to the doctor and received a prescription for one of the sulphur-based drugs...On one occasion during the summer, when I realized another infection was coming on, I took ten drops of stabilized oxygen in an eight ounce glass of water before going to bed, rather than taking the prescription drug. In spite of the discomfort, I was able to go to sleep and I awoke the next morning without a trace of the bladder problem.
M.M., NY U.S.A.

- My son Jon brought me a couple of bottles of stabilized oxygen when he came home for Christmas. The last four years I have been in the hospital 34 times, not counting the times I just went to the E.R. I've had angioplasty 12 times and I didn't have the energy to even do my housework. The last time I was in the hospital was just before Christmas. When I take stabilized oxygen for my angina, I feel better very quickly. I was on oxygen for a long time. Because of stabilized oxygen, now I don't have to carry an oxygen tank with me and I can go places I've not been able to go to in a long time. Best of all, I haven't had any chest pain for three months!I'm sending you a picture taken a few months ago. I will be 76 years old Friday and I feel like a spring chicken thanks to stabilized oxygen. Even the age spots on my hands and arms are clear now that I have been putting stabilized oxygen on them.
H.R., AZ U.S.A.

- My husband had an ugly mole on the back of his leg for 10 years. It was about 1/2 inch across. Lately, it had begun to turn strange colors and puff out about 1/8th of an inch, so now it was catching on his pants when he put them on and removed them. This caused tearing and bleeding. We were getting quite concerned about the negative change in this mole. We tried everything we could think of, but nothing worked. We even tried colloidal silver, but there was no improvement. Then we tried the new stabilized oxygen. The results were definitely worth sharing. We put the stabilized oxygen on a cotton ball and secured it over the mole

with a Band-Aid. We resaturated the cotton about 3 times a day - morning, after work, and bedtime. The first week, absolutely nothing happened. The second week, it started to turn even more colors and to dry up. The third week, it just fell off! After all these years -- end of mole, end of story. I'm sharing this because I would like to help others who might be considering freezing, cutting, or burning off such a nuisance and potential cancer problems. Try stabilized oxygen first. You might also be pleasantly surprised!
LS., WA U.S.A.

• My husband has suffered with asthma so severe that it was classified as "life-threatening · -- the most dreaded category in which to land. He was totally steroid dependent in order to control it. We lived in an area of North Carolina that was full of industrial pollution, and the problem was further aggravated by massive amounts of pollens of all kinds drifting in from the Blue Ridge Parkway. We also learned that we can put it directly into the nostrils and use it like nose drops, or fill a nasal spray bottle and spray up the nose. It relieves congestion and the often resulting sinus infection that can cause an overabundance of mucous. He always used to carry a nasal spray bottle to help him keep breath ing, but no longer. Another thing we learned as we shared our experience, is that we can fill a spray bottle and spray the stabilized oxygen toward the back of the throat and inhale. His Prednisone is now down to 3 mg per day, and considering that he was at 100 mg., you can imagine how grateful we are!
D. C., WA U.S.A.

• For 3 years I couldn't have any air blowing on me. I wore a heavy coat summer and winter. I couldn't use my air conditioner. It gets 95 here for four months in the summer. I was given a bottle of your stabilized oxygen. In one week's time I was better. In 2 weeks I was completely healed. Also my arthritis is much better. I tried every vitamin that they sell. Nothing helped. I took 20 drops morning and noon. I am 84 years old. I can't thank you enough for your stabilized oxygen.
R.P., TX U.S.A.

• I am a retired accountant, and for a long time I have suffered with severe pain in my elbows, forearms and shoulders. About four months ago I started taking stabilized oxygen. I started at 20 drops 2 times a day, and had no results. Then I increased it to 30 drops 3 times a day, in water. I experienced dramatic relief, and so I kept it at this level for 6 weeks. Then I decided to see if I could get the same results without using so much, so I dropped it to 20 drops 3 times a day, and still had the same results. So now I take 20 drops per day and am still doing just fine. I guess I just had to use a bit more to get enough in my system after years of being oxygen de-

prived. I have also dramatically reduced my medications for asthma by using the stabilized oxygen...I no longer need Prednisone. The year before I discovered your products I was in the hospital five times, and I have had no doubts that would land me there since being blessed with these formulas. Being a senior citizen, you can't imagine how grateful I am that you have helped me save my breath, my health, and my money! Thank you.
L.T., WI U.S.A.

- From earliest childhood, I have had every form of bronchial problems. After using stabilized oxygen, I am off antibiotics and inhalers. I am feeling much better with additional energy. I would recommend stabilized oxygen to anyone with any form of bronchial problems.
J.G., LA U.S.A.

- In July I started taking 20 drops of stabilized oxygen three times a day. Here are the results so far: After 4 days the cramps in my legs and feet stopped. Also the soles of my feet stopped burning. After six days my eyes were clear of burning and itching...After five days my stomach cramps disappeared. After seven days -- I've had manic depression for 30 years. With lithium, sometimes I have a few flashes of fantasy. It is gone. After seven days -- I've had emphysema for 13 years. My breathing has improved, both day and night and I have no pain. After seven days -- my stool has become normal. The best in 10 years -- frequency, substance, and ease. After 16 days the occasional problems I've had with my prostate have disappeared ...After 21 days, no pain or joint restriction to any bone. After three weeks I feel like a new man.
M.S., TX U.S.A.

- A year and a half ago my doctors prescribed thyroid medication. Soon after I started taking this medicine, I developed a bad cough. I believe I may be allergic to the medicine, but three different doctors I consulted told me to keep on taking it. So for the past year and a half I have been coughing everyday. I'm so happy I found stabilized oxygen! In less than a week my coughing stopped. I took 10 drops three times a day to start. Now I only have to take 10 drops a day and no more coughing! Thank You.
E.R., FL U.S.A.

- I was born with food allergies and so it came as no surprise when I got asthma after eating a small pat of butter that kept me out of school for three weeks. So I began with health problems and they multiplied. Chronic fatigue ... Headaches ... Sinus, were some of the things I suffered from, but the worst part was a feeling of terrible fatigue. My fatigue was worse

after eating. It felt like someone hit me in the pit of the stomach and knocked all my air out. Then I would have to lie down for a while until I recovered. After getting my first bottle of stabilized oxygen I took 21 drops and waited to see what would happen. WOW!! I could breathe through my nose!I thought it was just to hold my glasses. What a difference! I have ENERGY. Before everything was very hard to do, so much so that even after taking a shower, I had to lie down to catch my breath. Now I feel human again. I now walk two miles to the grocery store each day. It used to take me an hour - now just 40 minutes. I still have plenty of energy so sometimes we go to the mall shopping till 9 PM when they close. I'm walking 105 steps a minute and feel GREAT! I'm 68 on the way to 100.
K.E.H., UT U.S.A.

- I took 10 drops of stabilized oxygen twice the first day it came and I woke up the next morning pain free for the first time in a few years. I am going to keep on taking it, as it is such a relief to be pain free. Now I can shop and do things my painful back and hips never let me do before. I actually spent a whole day Christmas shopping this year. And I was able to do things the next day.
E.B., U.S.A.

- I took a 3 1/2 hour flight from Detroit to Phoenix in December. When I arrived in Phoenix, a severe headache hit me as I walked up the ramp. I believe that this was due to the lack of oxygen and fresh air during the flight and therefore my body needed oxygen! I carried a bottle of stabilized oxygen with me and put about 50 drops under my tongue and after 30 seconds washed it down with some water. Within three minutes the headache went away as fast as it came on. I gave my body what it needed.
J.E. U.S.A.

- My sister received a newsletter on stabilized oxygen. We were both trying to find something to help our Dad who was battling numerous health difficulties and on an inhaler and bedridden most of the time. I started Dad on stabilized oxygen, 30 drops twice a day. He is no longer on the inhaler. By the second dose of stabilized oxygen I had more energy. After four days the intense pain left my thighs, hips and arms and has not returned. I believe my body was full of toxic poison from undigested food that got in my blood.
L. G., MO U.S.A.

- I use stabilized oxygen twice a day and it keeps me off the breathing machine. If I miss using it for a day or two then I realize how much it helps. Then I start wheezing and am more short-breathed and can't do as much.

W.B. U.S.A.

- After taking stabilized oxygen for several months (20 to 30 drops per day), I find I have more energy and stamina, have become immune to colds and flu and the people in the office plus my family comment on how good I look and they are surprised to discover I'm almost 69. That's wonderful for the ego!

J. C., TX U.S.A.

- In March of 1997 I had a diagnosis of cancer in both lungs. I was told that surgery was the only solution because neither chemotherapy nor radiation were an acceptable option, because of my poor condition. I had some emphysema and a plugged main artery in my heart, and they weren't sure I'd make it through surgery. If I did nothing, I wouldn't live any more than six months to a year. I told them if I was going to die, I was going to die whole. In August I went fishing in Canada with my two sons and my youngest grandson. While sitting and talking one evening all of a sudden I pitched forward and was not breathing and had no heart beat. My youngest son gave me CPR while the oldest went to call an ambulance. Our grandson Casey PRAYED. In the hospital they found I had very low blood potassium, down to 2.5. For 30 hours they gave me potassium intravenously. After leaving the hospital I was very weak and staggering all over. I used a cane for about a month. One day, while seeing my chiropractor, he told me he had just read an article and the first person he though of was me. I asked him what it was. He said stabilized oxygen. I asked at several health food stores and none had heard of it. Finally my chiropractor got some in and I was there when it came. Three days after starting the stabilized oxygen I threw my cane away. In November we went to Arizona to our park and I bought myself a bicycle. No one had expected to see me back...Now every day someone comes to my door because of how I look and act, wanting some of this stabilized oxygen. I take 30 drops 3 or 4 times a day and no medications. I take other vitamins and minerals, but I never leave home without stabilized oxygen. In December the x-rays showed that both tumors were getting smaller. This is a long way from the doc tor telling me to get into the hospice program in August.

H.C.L. U.S.A.

- In January of 1968, when I was 41 years old, I suffered a massive embolism of the lungs. After weeks in the hospital I went home, but I have never been able to do much of anything since then. After 10 minutes or so I have always had to stop and rest. I never could hurry or run or walk upstairs without stopping and resting. Now with taking a few drops of stabilized oxygen about 3 times a day, I am a different person.

M.G. U.S.A.

- My husband George, who is 96 years old, has clogged arteries in his legs. This has bothered him for several years. He could walk only about 100 feet, then stop, because of the severe pain in the muscles in his calves and thighs. After a few minutes rest he could walk another 100 feet or so. Our doctor said this was happening because the muscles were not getting the oxygen they needed due to the clogged blood vessels. We tried many supplements, but nothing happened. When I read about stabilized oxygen in a newsletter, I sent for it. I gave my husband 18 drops in 7 ounces of bottled spring water, twice a day, before breakfast and a half-hour before dinner. It took three months to be effective. Now he can walk a half-mile, sit for 10 minutes to rest and then walk back home without pain. My husband also has severe arthritis in the low er spine due to a bad fall on icy pavement four years ago. He no longer complains of the pain and he stands and walks straighter since taking stabilized oxygen. P.S. We have been married 72 years. (I am 87 years old.)

A.I., NJ U.S.A.

- I have been taking stabilized oxygen for six months. It has improved my life 98%. I have had chronic bronchitis since 1962 (36 years!). I coughed most of the time. Since being on the stabilized oxygen, I no longer cough. It's a miracle! I am 68 years young. I thank the Lord every day for stabilized oxygen.

D.S., FL U.S.A.

- I used stabilized oxygen on my husband's diabetic ulcers (sores) on his foot and within two and a half weeks they were all healed up, whereas no doctor could get them to heal. As for myself, I use 15 to 30 drops in water each day. I noticed I can go up and down stairs much better than before. Also a lump I had on my neck below my back skull is gone. Now I can turn my head better. Also my neighbor thinks there is nothing better for cuts and scratches.

R.H., UT U.S.A.

- For several years, my 10-year-old granddaughter had a warty area in the web between two fingers, which interfered with daily use of her hand. Various home treatments included drugstore remedies, trimming, hydrogen peroxide, aloe gel, aromatherapy oils and minerals solutions, but nothing was completely successful. It eventually became the size of a nickel. Her pediatrician said it was "the worst kind of wart" and used Histofreeze on it. Still, it returned. Then dermatologists cut it out and used liquid nitrogen - all of this involving pain and extensive recovery time. Still the wart returned! She then I began to rub stabilized oxygen on it twice a

day, and the skin became normal in one month. She is careful to keep an eye on the area, and still uses the stabilized oxygen several times a week for prevention. Personally, I rub stabilized oxygen on those horrid age spots, and find that they lighten.
J.R., NH U.S.A.

- I'm really pleased with the results I've had in using stabilized oxygen for "dry eyes!" I'm finally rid of this irritating condition after two and a half years. When I feel it coming on I take 20 drops under the tongue and within minutes it's gone. Great Product!
J.H, ID U.S.A.

- I reached my 89th birthday on February 20, 1998. I was born with a "shunt" (a hole) in my heart and am the only person so afflicted to live beyond 50 years. The New England Medical Journal will confirm. I had moderate emphysema (from smoking for 71 years), an enlarged heart, and problems with my bronchial tubes and pulmonary arteries. I have been taking stabilized oxygen...twice a day for 6 months and have experienced sensational assistance. I walk briskly and can sing like a lark!
S.S., FL U.S.A.

- Your stabilized oxygen is indeed amazing. I have an allergy to smog, and get severe ear infections ...My allergy to smog was severe enough to cause a brain hemorrhage 30 years ago, and I had to move more than once, to elude the smog. With stabilized oxygen, I can stay where I am and enjoy daily living.
F.B., CA U.S.A.

- My mother was suddenly diagnosed with severe blockage of the main arteries and doctors would not operate due to the possible consequences of such an operation. Soon my mother was bed-ridden to the point where she could not even get out of her room because she was too fatigued and tired and in need of her oxygen tank. Then I found out about stabilized oxygen. I sent a supply to her and in three days she was up on her own, no more oxygen tank, running errands, cooking just like normal.
W.G., CA U.S.A.

- When I read that stabilized oxygen removes seborrhea from the scalp it was almost too good to believe. I have had seborrhea all my adult life. I took 30 drops of stabilized oxygen in pure water three times a day between meals. The very first week the awful stuff cleared up. I keep taking it in smaller amounts now.
E.P., OR U.S.A.

- I work at an astronomical observatory on top of Mauna Kea, here in Hawaii. There is only 60% of the oxygen normally found at sea-level. I had read about stabilized oxygen, so a few months ago, I ordered three bottles... and started using it daily. I take about twice the recommended dosage. I notice a definite increase in energy, mental clarity, and ability to perform strenuous tasks at this high altitude. I have not noticed any negative side effects.
J.C., HI U.S.A.

- After biopsy surgery on September 25, 1997, the miasma and surrounding area were not healing as well as I hoped. After five months, there was a mass under the skin. The incision was dark red and Vitamin E seemed to heal it only so far. There was frequent discomfort and pain. I began to apply stabilized oxygen to the area in March. The discomfort decreased after just a couple of applications. The scar resumed healing. Two months later, the mass has greatly diminished in size...the scar is smaller. I can also testify to the effects of ingesting the stabilized oxygen. On the treadmill, I could only walk about 7 minutes, with stabilized oxygen, I walk 20 minutes!
I.S., AZ U.S.A.

- Stabilized oxygen has been wonderful for me. I've been taking 15 drops twice a day for several months now. My thinking has never been clearer and my in tuition has sharpened greatly so that I'm seeing things more clearly and making better decisions. I'm also sleeping better and the content of my dreams doesn't drag me down anymore.
M.W., CA U.S.A.

- Stabilized oxygen makes me feel so good! It reminds me of the Miracle Grow I give my plants, but this stabilized oxygen is for me!
D.P., NM U.S.A.

- I bought a bottle of stabilized oxygen just to see if it would work. I have had headaches for more than fifteen years. It is caused by a benign tumor behind my right ear. No operations of any kind, says the doctor. He has tried all kinds of medicines, no cure. I put 25 drops of stabilized oxygen in a glass, poured some distilled water into the glass and stirred it with a plastic spoon. Bingo, two hours later my headache was gone. I can even see better, and my hearing is a little better too.
W.F., NC U.S.A.

- My father who is 76 years old had gotten a very bad chest cold. He felt so weak he wouldn't have any visitors. I gave him a bottle of stabilized oxygen and after a week he was back to his old self. He takes it every day

now. My husband has a friend that had emphysema and he got tired just walking up or down stairs. My husband told him about stabilized oxygen and the man bought some. He called about three weeks later and said it was working very good for him - so much so that he now walks about seven blocks a day and feels great.
L.B., PA U.S.A.

• It seems incredible that just 40 little drops of stabilized oxygen in a glass of water daily has made me a new woman! I feel completely renewed in body and mind and also uplifted in spirit. At 84 years old, I live life enthusiastically and joyfully, looking forward to each day's tasks as well as rewards. I'm in close touch with, and adore my two grown children and my grandchildren. Frequently I play winning bridge at my club, so obviously this keeps me mentally alert. So, what more could one want!
M.W., FL U.S.A.

• I had a burn, 1⁄2 inch by 1 1⁄4 inch, on my hand from touching the hot oven rack. It had been there for approximately two years. It would scab over and then peel, leaving a redness, sometimes to the point of almost bleeding. One day when I was taking stabilized oxygen internally, I put a drop on this area. After putting a drop on daily for about 5 days the area was noticeably healing. Another 2 days and there was only a very light area of redness; only noticeable to myself.
Dr. S.C., MA U.S.A.

• I cannot in all honesty say enough about what stabilized oxygen has done for me. I had a touch of emphysema and had to use two inhalers three times a day and I used to wheeze also. Then I took stabilized oxygen to see if it would work and found to my amazement that it did! I felt really good and had a sense of well being that I hadn't had in years. I found I needn't depend on my inhalers anymore and my wheeze went away. I could breathe again like I used to. Thank you for stabilized oxygen.
G.C., TX U.S.A.

• I have been using stabilized oxygen for six months now and have lots of energy. It clears up cuts in no time. My husband is 77 and is diabetic. He uses it every day also and has lots of energy. Plus it cleaned up the ulcers on his feet which no doctor could do. It's a wonderful product which we will never be without.
R.H., UT U.S.A.

• I want to say thank you for letting me know about stabilized oxygen. It sure is great and I sure do feel super. It got rid of the gas I've had for a

long time. Of course I've been on vitamins for years, but stabilized oxygen is the best. I hope I never run out of it. I don't ache in my joints as before. I sure love it. I also give it to my husband. He has a chemical imbalance and by taking it he is much better.
F.P., MA U.S.A.

• I tried stabilized oxygen to see if it did everything that it was claimed it could do. I have fibromyalgia and one of the most annoying problems is a "fuzzy" brain. Stabilized oxygen has given me a much clearer brain function, more energy and has lessened my pain. My husband has COPD and the stabilized oxygen has eased his breathing difficulties so he can be more comfortable.
A.G., NC U.S.A.

• I take 20 drops of stabilized oxygen each morning. Recently I had a breaking out of running sores on my right hand. Some of the remedies I tried without success were hydrocortisone, Benadryl, comfrey poultices, Vitamin E, sulfur and lard, and potassium per manganate. I started using stabilized oxygen every three hours and my hand is now doing very well. The itching and weeping have gone away.
E.R., MI U.S.A.

• Stabilized oxygen has relieved the pain and redness of my right hand. Before starting to use stabilized oxygen I was rubbing my hand in pain medicine and wearing gloves at night. I no longer wear the gloves. My breathing is much better and this allergy season has not been rough by using stabilized oxygen. I have more energy and am able to do more as my arthritis pains are not like before.
H.C., WV U.S.A.

• Thank you for your product stabilized oxygen. It has given me back my life. Four years ago I suffered a heart attack brought on by severe asthma. The past four years have been spent searching and trying every product I could find. Some helped, most didn't. I heard of stabilized oxygen from a friend. Now after two bottles and one month I am living again! The chest pains are gone. The asthma is now a rare occurrence. I look forward to taking stabilized oxygen every day of my life. It has made such a difference. Life is now exciting and wonderful again.
K.D., CA U.S.A.

• I have been taking stabilized oxygen for about three months. I am diabetic and before I started taking stabilized oxygen my legs used to hurt very bad when I walked. My legs stopped hurting the day after I started taking stabilized oxygen and have not hurt me since. My wife has intro-

duced our neighbors to it, and they also have had positive results. I live in an elderly housing project and all the people here are either elderly or disabled.
J.H., HI U.S.A.

- Stabilized oxygen - what a fantastic product! After taking it, I now don't need my Claritin and Vancanase A.Q. for my asthma. I had asthma for six years and this is the best I have felt in ten years! Stabilized oxygen also heals cuts. Four weeks ago I had a cut, bad enough for stitches. I put some stabilized oxygen on it and the cut is now almost gone.
D.M., PA U.S.A.

- I was disabled last October with lung cancer...I could not walk 50 paces without stopping. My breath and legs would give out. I read about stabilized oxygen and decided to get some. I have taken it for about four months. It's a Godsend. My legs don't give out any more; my breathing is 25% better. My blood pressure also dropped. I feel so much better. I don't even think of my condition. I'm telling everyone about stabilized oxygen.
I.W., WV U.S.A.

- I have heart disease. I am undergoing alternative therapy (chelation), in addition to taking various supplements. Stabilized oxygen has made a large difference in controlling my angina. I am able to reduce it or even prevent it. I am recommending stabilized oxygen to anyone suffering from respiratory or cardiovascular problems. I find I get the fastest relief when taking the stabilized oxygen sublingually.
Dr. U.B., MI U.S.A.

- I want to take a few lines to praise that wonderful stabilized oxygen you make available. I had originally purchased it for myself to aid me in this pollen season here in Ohio. When I first received it I was fairly "stuffed up" in my sinuses. After 7 or 8 drops I waited patiently hoping to see some difference, any difference in maybe 5 or 6 hours or even the next day. I was pleasantly shocked to find that in just a few minutes (about 5) my breathing was normal again. I was truly ecstatic. That night I placed the bottle of stabilized oxygen by my bed in case I needed some during the night. By around 6 AM my son (who is 5 years old) came to me and said "Mommy, Mommy, I can't breathe !" The stabilized oxygen came to my mind and I gave him 5 drops under his tongue. It worked even quicker on him (about 2 minutes). Now when he wakes up and his nose is stuffed he just asks me for the stabilized oxygen. I've also given the stabilized oxygen to my 80 year old Dad when my parents visited us recently. Since their visit was 2 weeks long, I thought it would be a perfect opportunity to give some "life" back to my Dad. You see, Dad has a history of heart problems and has

been very weak and out of breath. Dad noticed a difference in the first day. By day 5 he was riding my Schwinn Airdyne Exercise bike for 5 minutes with its oscillating handle bars.
N.W., OH U.S.A.

- I have been a diabetic for over 22 years and have always had a problem with my vision. After taking stabilized oxygen for just a short time, my vision has improved tremendously. I am very pleased with the results.
L.F.T., AL U.S.A.

- My husband has diabetes and his leg used to hurt him so much when he walked. But since he has been taking stabilized oxygen, all of the pain has gone. His sugar count is great. He feels great. Now where he works, they all want to start taking the stabilized oxygen. I can only say that this is the best thing he has ever taken to help him.
L.H., HI U.S.A.

- In 1996 and 1997 I was very short of breath all the time. My oxygen level would get in the low 80's and I felt BLAH!I have had asthma all my life, and was always using inhalers, pills galore, and going to the doctor every month. My diabetes was in bad shape. My sugar count was always in the 300 range, and got as high as 600. I took insulin shots, and medication and the level got down in the 180 to 200 count range. In early 1998 I heard about stabilized oxygen. I ordered two bottles. After 90 days I had my oxygen level tested, and it was 97%. My oxygen level stays in the mid to high 90% range. Today my blood sugar count is in the 90 to 120 range, depending on my diet. My oxygen stays in the high 90% range, and I take no medication of any kind. I am 70 years old. I wish I had known about stabilized oxygen 25 years ago. Now I can enjoy hunting, fishing and gardening without shortness of breath and wheezing like a winded horse. I haven't been to the doctor in 5 months. I am a firm believer in stabilized oxygen. Presently I am taking 30 drops twice a day in a small amount of water, then drinking a glass of water following the small amount of water with stabilized oxygen. I have lost 25 pounds the past year and I'm feeling great!
H.V. U.S.A.

- I am 70 years old and have tried many products with no perceivable befits. I only have a small Social Security pension and it is difficult to buy all the nutrients I am told I should be taking. I have been unable to take a deep breath for several years. I have practiced for some time forcing air into my lower lungs 20 times, then forcing it into my upper lungs 20 times, but I could not get it into both parts at the same time, and could not get the air into the very top of my lungs. After taking stabilized oxygen for

one month, I woke up the next morning and took a deep breath and filled my lungs with air, clear to the top! Now I practice taking dee breaths several times a day.
P.D., OR U.S.A.

- I have read many of the testimonials of people using stabilized oxygen. Nowhere did I see an example of simply rubbing the stabilized oxygen on painful are as. I tried this with an arthritic joint of mine and the pain stopped instantly! I couldn't believe it!
R.C., NY U.S.A.

- I thought I would share with you the best piece of news in the whole world. I am a 56 year old woman and have been hooked on nasal spray since I was 28. Not just any spray but the strongest 4-way Menthol. None others would work. I used two to three bottles a week. I have been using stabilized oxygen for about 3 weeks. Yesterday it occurred to me that I didn't use the 4-way even once and last night I used a saline moisturizing spray one time. Today I didn't use it again. This is a miracle! The E.N.T. I saw a few years ago told me that I would never get off nose spray. Thanks a million. Never stop making stabilized oxygen. It is incredible. It has also been helping my husband's lung problems.
J.S., ID U.S.A.

- I was developing a cataract in my left eye. I decided that if stabilized oxygen is safe to take by mouth it surely could not harm my eye. Imagine my amazement when the second day of using a drop twice daily I could tell a difference. I have now finished my first bottle and my problem is almost totally gone. Thank you for stabilized oxygen.
E.P., CA U.S.A.

- How can I say 'Thank You?" You have given back my life! Nearly five years ago, I became very ill and suffered debilitating pain and fatigue. After several months of expensive testing I was diagnosed with lupus, possible co-mingled with scleroderma: two incurable, potentially fatal diseases. I was 24 years old. We began aggressive treatment of my symptoms, and I gained a measure of relief, but was still unable to work a job or give my family 100%. I still suffered from constant pain and bouts of severe fatigue. Then about six weeks ago, my grandmother introduced me to stabilized oxygen, and my whole life changed. Here a few of the things that have changed: I sleep soundly without being awakened by pain; I wake up refreshed and energized; my photo-sensitivity has improved dramatically; the dark circles under my eyes are gone; I put in 16-18 hour days and don't spend two weeks in bed recovering; I have energy to do

things I thought I would never do again; the constant pain I have lived with the five years has lessened considerably; I am now working full-time plus going to college two nights a week, plus taking care of two young children. I would never do it without stabilized oxygen. From the bottom of my heart, I thank you!
N.C., FL U.S.A.

- I have been taking stabilized oxygen for about two years now. It helps keep Candida under control...By the way, I am 83 years old.
V.S., CA U.S.A.

- I wish I had known about stabilized oxygen years ago. I started taking stabilized oxygen ...about three months ago. I am 86 years old. I could hardly get out of bed from back pain. I also had lots of pain in my right shoulder. It was so bad I couldn't raise my arm to comb my hair. I am much better now.
Y.H., CA U.S.A.

- Stabilized oxygen - what a product. Everything you need in one little bottle. It has really changed my life. I now have energy to keep up with all the young guys at work. And even beat them at pole top rescue. (I work for the electric company.)
J.H., CO U.S.A.

- I am 80 years of age and have terrible lungs and was having asthma attacks day and night for a long time. I received some literature about stabilized oxygen about five months ago and I ordered four bottles and have been taking it since that time. Am I a believer? I swear I have not had even one attack since starting on it. I was on Theodurr and Albuterol inhalers. Three inhalers per month. Now I have almost forgotten about Theodurr and inhalers...
I.D., LA U.S.A.

- I have had blocked arteries for a long time. I also have emphysema and lung disease. The doctors told me that my left lung was the size of a 12 or 13 year old and my right lung was not working at 100%. The pain in my chest would put me back in the hospital again and again...I have not had any more chest pain at all.
C.B., NC U.S.A.

- Stabilized oxygen has worked wonders. After using it for two months I noticed a profound difference in my breathing. I am so grateful that I discovered such a worry-free and simple remedy, helping me with my hay fever.

A.S., FL U.S.A.

- I had seven surgeries to remove tumors in the bladder. But my May 27, 1998 the doctor said there was nothing more he could do but remove the bladder. I talked with my family doctor and he suggested a second opinion. At my age, 85, I didn't see how I could go through the surgery of removing the bladder. This is when I ordered ...stabilized oxygen. Three months later the doctor took a scope and found five small tumors, which he removed ...
O.F., OH U.S.A.

- Of all the vitamins I have taken, and still do, none has produced the miraculous changes that stabilized oxygen has done for me. I have only been taking it for a short time, but already I can tell the difference. I use to be very unsteady when I walked, today it is as if I had taken 20 years off my age. I used to awaken two or three times every night, short of breath, it was frightening. Now I have perfect rest. Truly, I can't say nearly enough in praise of this wonderful stabilized oxygen.
LP., NV U.S.A.

- I'm 66 years old and every day after lunch, I would take a little rest. Now after taking stabilized oxygen I don't feel I need to take an afternoon nap anymore.
R.R.S., WA U.S.A.

- In 1997 I found I had Myelo Dysplastic Syndrome. It is a rare condition of faulty red blood cells causing anemia. I have been taking stabilized oxygen for one year and I feel better than last year. My eyesight also seems to be getting better. I take 30 drops four times a day and when I feel tired I take 10 drops by mouth. I believe this is keeping me going.
J.M., OH U.S.A.

- My wife has advanced Alzheimers. I have been giving her an average of 30 drops twice a day. There is some indication that is doing some good, so I will continue to order more. I have started to take it myself and feel it is cleansing the colon and giving me more energy.
W.W., OH U.S.A.

- I am 64 years old and had been a caretaker for many years. It left me drained and without energy. I also en countered some health problems in the last 2 years. I took other vitamins but they did not work well...In the state of health I was in it took about 3-4 weeks to feel a difference. However, since then I will not be without it ever again. Now at least I feel better than I have felt in some time. My general health has improved and I

am able to walk better without the constant aches and pains from arthritis.
M.G., NY U.S.A.

- Stabilized oxygen has helped me in several ways. Taking it before bedtime keeps my sinuses open for the night. It is also helping my kidney problem and I am gaining in strength. It is a very valuable vitamin.
V. M., MS U.S.A.

The testimonials in this appendix contain, for the most part, unverified results that have been forwarded to us by users of stabilized oxygen dietary supplements, and may not reflect the typical user's experience, may not apply to the average person and are not intended to represent nor guarantee that anyone will achieve the same or similar results.

Results described by a researcher or medical professional, or other reputable third party sources, should infer that the typical results as stated are more reliable than consumer testimonials. However, you should always perform due diligence and never take such results at face value.

The author is not responsible for any errors or omissions in typical results information supplied to him by researchers, medical professionals or other reputable third parties.

It is possible, that even with perfect use of stabilized oxygen dietary supplements, you will not achieve the results described in testimonials. These testimonials are meant to showcase the typical results using stabilized oxygen, and should not be taken as the results a typical user will get.

APPENDIX FIVE:
Uses for Ozone[199]

> You wouldn't believe how many FDA officials or relatives or acquaintances of FDA officials come to see me as patients in Hanover...or directors of the AMA, or ACA, or the presidents of orthodox cancer institutes. That's the fact.
> Hans Nieper[200]

The first report of ozone being used to purify blood in test tubes was by the German Dr. C. Lender in **1870**.

The first ozone generators were developed by Werner von Siemens in Germany in **1857**.

The first American therapeutic use of ozone was by Dr. John H. Kellogg in ozone steam saunas at his Battle Creek, Michigan sanitarium from **1880**.

In **1885**, the Florida Medical Association published "Ozone" by Dr. Charles J. Kenworthy, MD, detailing the use of ozone for therapeutic purposes.

In October **1893**, the world's first water treatment plant using ozone was installed in Ousbaden, Holland.[201]

In September **1896**, Nikola Tesla patented his first ozone generator, and in **1900** he formed the Tesla Ozone Co. Tesla sold ozone machines and ozonated olive oil to doctors for medical use.

In **1898**, the Institute for Oxygen Therapy Healing was started in Berlin by Thauerkauf and Luth. They experimented with injecting ozone.

Ozone was bonded to magnesium in a catalytic process to produce Homozon by Dr. Eugene Blass in **1898**.

Beginning in **1898**, Dr. Benedict Lust, a German doctor practicing

---

[199] From: http://www.envirohealthtech.com/oxidative_history.htm

[200] Hans Alfred Nieper (23 May 1928 – 21 October 1998) was a controversial German alternative medicine practitioner who devised "Nieper Therapy". He is best known for his claims to be able to treat cancer, multiple sclerosis, and other serious diseases using ozone and other natural therapies.

[201] Today there are more than 3,000 municipalities around the world that use ozone to clean and treat water and sewage,

in New York, established the practice of Naturopathy, based on ozone therapy.

In **1898**, homeopathic Dr. S.R. Beckwith, of New York, published his booklet describing the use of his invention, the Thermo-Ozone Generator, in the treatment of a wide variety of diseases.

In **1902**, J.H. Clarke's "A Dictionary of Practical Materia Medica", London, describes the successful use of ozonated water ("Oxygenium") in treating anemia, cancer, diabetes, influenza, morphine poisoning, canker sores, strychnine poisoning and whooping cough.

In **1904**, "The Medical Uses of Hydrozone (ozonated water) and Glycozone (ozonated olive oil) by Charles Marchand, a New York chemist appeared in its 19th edition. The book remains in the Library of Congress with the U.S. Surgeon General's stamp of approval on it.[202]

In **1911**, "A Working Manual of High Frequency Currents" was published by Dr. Noble Eberhart, MD, the head of the Department of Physiologic Therapeutics at Loyola University, Chicago. In Chapter 9, he details the use of ozone to treat tuberculosis, anemia, chlorosis, tinnitus, whooping cough, asthma, bronchitis, hay fever, insomnia, pneumonia, diabetes, gout and syphilis.

In **1912**, Dr. H.C. Bennett published "Electro-Therapeutic Guide". He described the use of Ozol, ozone gas breathed after running it through eucalyptus, pine or thyme oils.

In **1913**, the Eastern Association for Oxygen Therapy was formed by Dr. Eugene Blass and other German associates.

During World War I, (**1914-1918**) ozone was used to treat wounds, trench foot, gangrene and the effects of poison gas.

In **1915**, Dr. Albert Wolff of Berlin used ozone to treat colon cancer, cervical cancer and decubitus ulcers.

In **1920**, Dr. Charles Neiswanger, MD, President of the Chicago Hospital College of Medicine, published "Electro Therapeutical Practice". Chapter 32 was entitle "Ozone as a Therapeutic Agent".

In the **1920**s, Nikola Tesla allowed the licensed production of his ozone air purifier in Canada which was based on his cold plasma design.

---

[202] This active use of therapeutic ozone predates the establishment of the FDA in 1906 and therefore many believe this qualifies ozone therapy to be grandfathered into acceptance as a medical modality by the FDA in spite of the FDA's refusal to do so.

In **1929**, a book called "Ozone and Its Therapeutic Action" was published in the U.S. listing 114 diseases and how to treat all of them with ozone. Its 40 authors were the heads of all the leading American hospitals.

In **1930**, the Swiss dentist Dr. E. A. Fisch used ozone in dentistry, and published many papers on its use. He also introduced ozone to the the distinguished Austrian surgeon, Dr. Erwin Payr in **1932**.

In **1933**, the American Medical Association (AMA), headed by Morris Fishbein, attempted to eliminate all medical treatments that were competitive to drug therapies. The suppression of ozone therapy in the U.S. began in this year and continues to this day. Only ten U.S. states protect doctors from prosecution by state laws. At the request of the AMA, the FDA began seizing generators in the **1940**s and consents to do so in states that do not have laws on the books to protect doctors from using ozone treatments.

Dr. Aubourg and Dr. Lacoste were French physicians using ozone insufflation[203] **1934-1938**. Aubourg wrote "Medical Ozone: Production, Dosage and Methods of Clinical Application" in **1938**. He gave ozone rectally, vaginally, injected into wounds and used it by allowing patients to breathe it. In his 8,000 recorded applications of ozone treatments, there were no harmful side effects.

In **1935**, M. Sourdeau published a paper on "Ozone in Therapy" in France.

Dr. Hans Wolff wrote the book "Medical Ozone" in the **1940**s.

In **1942**, "Gordon Detoxification and Hydro Surgery: Theory and Practice" was published covering the medical uses of ozone as colon cleanser.

During World War II, (**1939-1945**) Dr. Robert Mayer, M.D. learned about ozone therapy from German prisoners of war at Ellis Island, and used ozone in his practice for the next 45 years.

In **1948**, Dr. William Turska of Oregon began using an ozone machine of his own design (Aethozone). In 1951, Dr. Turska wrote the article "Oxidation", which is still used as a reference article today.

In **1953**, the German physician, Dr. Hans Wolff, began training doctors in the use of ozone therapy.

In **1954**, Frank Totney published "Oxygen : Master of Cancer".

---

[203] The act of blowing something (as a gas, powder, or vapor) into a body cavity.

In **1957**, Dr. J. Hansler patented an ozone generator which formed the basis of a revival of German-based ozone therapy. Today, over 8,000 German doctors use ozone therapy every day on patients.

In **1961**, the Encyclopedia of Chemical Technology stated: "During the 80 year history of the large scale usage of ozone, there has never been a human death attributed to it".

In **1971**, Dr. Hans Wolff and Prof. Dr. Siegfried Rilling founded The German Medical Society for Ozone Therapy.

In **1972**, The International Association for Oxygen Therapy was founded by Dr. George Freibott. this organization became the successor to the Eastern Association for Oxygen Therapy founded in 1913.

In **1977**, Dr. Renate Viebahn provided an overview of ozone's biological action.

In **1979**, Dr. George Freibott successfully treated a Haitian AIDS patient suffering Kaposi's sarcoma with ozone.

In **1980**, Dr. Horst Kief also reported success with ozone therapy for AIDS patients.

In **1980**, F. Sweet, et al, publish "Ozone Selectively Inhibits Human Cancer Cell Growth" in the peer-reviewed journal, Science, Vol. 209.

In **1982**, the German medical textbook "Medical Ozone" was published by Dr. E. Fischer Medical Publications in Heidelberg.

In **1983**, the first International Ozone Association medical conference was held, in Washington, D.C. The abstracts were published in the book "Medical Applications of Ozone", compiled and edited by Julius Laraus.

In **1985**, Dr. Renate Viebahn published "The Biochemical Process Underlying Ozone Therapy". that same year, Dr. Siegfried Rilling published "Basic Clinical Applications of Ozone Therapy".

In **1987**, Dr. Siegfried Rilling and Dr. Renate Viebahn collaborated on the publication of " The Use of Ozone in Medicine". This textbook is still considered the standard medical text on ozone application.

In **1988**, Dr. Gerard Sunnen at the Bellevue Medical Center in New York City, stated in an article entitled "Ozone in Medicine," that ozone was commonly used worldwide in treating herpes, AIDS, flu, wounds, burns, staph infections, fungal and radiation injuries, gangrene, colitis, fistula, hemorrhoids anal infections, virus infections, hepatitis, cancer, diabetes, arteriosclerosis, periodontal disease, intestinal and bladder inflammations. Ozone baths can be used to treat eczema and skin ulcers, ozone salve can treat skin ulcers and fungal growths.

In **1990**, the Cubans reported success in treating glaucoma, conjunctivitis and retinitis pigmentosa with ozone.

In **1992**, the Russians reported the successful use of ozone in a brine bath to treat burns.

In June **1994**, Plasmafire International sponsored an ozone symposium in Vancouver Canada. More than 160 professionals in all fields attended. A direct result of this conference was that ozone therapy is now recognized as an accepted modality by the Naturopathic Association of British Colombia and over 40 naturopaths now treat patients regularly with ozone therapy.

In **1994** Ed McCabe's book, "Oxygen Therapies," (republished in 2004 as "Flood your body with Oxygen") is published bringing the awareness of oxygen therapies to the mainstream population.

Today, after 150 years of usage and successful therapeutic results, ozone therapy is now officially recognized in Germany, Italy, France, Russia, Romania, Poland, Czech Republic, Hungary, Yugoslavia, Bulgaria, Israel, Japan, Singapore, Brazil, Cuba, Mexico, 4 Canadian provinces and 14 U.S. states (Alaska, Washington, California, Colorado, Nevada, New Mexico, Texas, Oklahoma, Georgia, New York, North Carolina, Ohio, Minnesota).

About the Author:

Stephen R. Krauss, Ph.D. has over 40 years of executive management experience in sales, manufacturing, and nutritional formulation and distribution on an international level. Dr. Krauss introduced Activated Stabilized Oxygen to the market in 1996 and, since then, he's established his company Oxigenesis as the world's leading formulator, manufacturer, and distributor of oxygen-enhanced health products. He has been a featured guest on nationally syndicated radio talk shows to educate on the topics of oxygen and holistic wellness. He has also worked as a national training consultant with Fortune 500 companies, state and federal government agencies and universities.

Dr. Krauss received his Undergraduate Degree in the Liberal Arts from California State Polytechnic University, with minors in Computer Science, Biology and Speech Communication. He has a Graduate Degree in Education with a Lifetime Secondary Teaching Credential, and an MBA and a Ph.D in International Business.